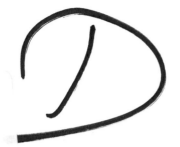

Coronary Heart Disease

YOUR QUESTIONS ANSWERED

For Elsevier

Commissioning Editor: Fiona Conn
Project Development Manager: Isobel Black
Project Manager: Frances Affleck
Design Direction: George Ajayi
Illustration Manager: Bruce Hogarth
Illustrator: Hardlines

Coronary Heart Disease

YOUR QUESTIONS ANSWERED

David E Newby
BA BSc (Hons) PhD BM DM FRCP
BHF Reader, University of Edinburgh
and Consultant Cardiologist
Royal Infirmary
Edinburgh, UK

John R Cockcroft
BSc MB ChB FRCP
Professor of Cardiology, Wales Heart
Research Institute
and Honorary Consultant Cardiologist
University Hospital of Wales
Cardiff, UK

Ian B Wilkinson
BM BCh MA DM MRCP
Lecturer in Clinical Pharmacology
The University of Cambridge
and Honorary Consultant Physician
Addenbrooke's Hospital NHS Trust
Cambridge, UK

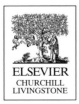

ELSEVIER
CHURCHILL
LIVINGSTONE

EDINBURGH LONDON NEW YORK OXFORD PHILADELPHIA ST LOUIS SYDNEY TORONTO 2005

ELSEVIER
CHURCHILL
LIVINGSTONE

Cover image © Simon Fraser/Science Photo Library

First published 2005

ISBN 0 4430 7464 X

British Library Cataloguing in Publication Data
A catalogue record for this book is available from the British Library

Library of Congress Cataloging in Publication Data
A catalog record for this book is available from the Library of Congress

Notice
Medical knowledge is constantly changing. Standard safety precautions must be followed, but as new research and clinical experience broaden our knowledge, changes in treatment and drug therapy may become necessary or appropriate. Readers are advised to check the most current product information provided by the manufacturer of each drug to be administered to verify the recommended dose, the method and duration of administration, and contraindications. It is the responsibility of the practitioner, relying on experience and knowledge of the patient, to determine dosages and the best treatment for each individual patient. Neither the Publisher nor the authors assume any liability for any injury and/or damage to persons or property arising from this publication.
The Publisher

your source for books,
journals and multimedia
in the health sciences

www.elsevierhealth.com

The
Publisher's
policy is to use
**paper manufactured
from sustainable forests**

Printed in China

Contents

Preface

Coronary heart disease (CHD) is one of the major causes of morbidity and mortality in the western world – death rates from CHD in the UK are amongst the highest in the world, with over 120 000 deaths per year. CHD is now the most common cause of premature death in the UK, accounting for 23% of premature deaths in men and 14% in women. The burden of CHD is also considerable in economic terms, costing the UK economy around £7 billion each year. Death rates from CHD have been falling over the past ten years and a recent government report (*The Boyle Report*, published March 2004) suggested that in individuals under the age of 65 'heart attacks are likely to become a thing of the past'. Much of this reduction in death rates from CHD over the past decade has been due to increases in the number of invasive procedures (for example coronary artery bypass grafting and angioplasty, which are reviewed in this book). In addition, improved pharmacological intervention with drugs, such as cholesterol-lowering statins and improved antithrombotic agents, again reviewed in this book, have contributed significantly to reduce death rates from CHD. However, reduced death rates from CHD, welcome though they are, do not accurately reflect the overall situation regarding CHD.

Currently over 2 million men and women in the UK are suffering from angina, the most common manifestation of CHD, and in addition 650 000 people have heart failure. Therefore, although mortality from CHD is definitely declining, morbidity is not. Indeed, the incidence of CHD may be set to rise dramatically due to the enormous increase in obesity and physical inactivity amongst the UK population. Obesity is a major risk factor for diabetes, a condition which significantly increases the risk of CHD and rates of obesity have tripled since the mid 1980s If this and other public health issues are not addressed as a matter of urgency, then it is quite possible that the incidence of CHD will actually rise, despite a fall in death rate.

Although secondary prevention of CHD has already made a significant contribution to a decrease in death rates, primary prevention of CHD must now be the focus of our efforts over the next decade. As the philosopher Erasmus said, 'prevention is better than cure'. It is also cheaper; indeed, heart disease costs the UK health care systems £2 billion annually, the hospital care of individuals with CHD accounting for over 50% of expenditure with less than 1% spent on prevention.

This book is written at a time which has seen significant increases in life expectancy in many developed countries, leading to new problems related to the normal vascular ageing process. Large arteries stiffen with age, thus increasing the risk of systolic hypertension, CHD and heart failure. Indeed, in individuals normotensive at the age of 55 years, the lifetime risk of developing systolic hypertension is 90%. In ageing societies, the boundaries between normal vascular ageing and disease are therefore becoming increasingly blurred and will require improved methods of risk stratification beyond those currently available, such as conventional sphygmomanometry. Such techniques, including non-invasive determination of arterial stiffness, have been recommended in the recent European Society of Hypertension Guidelines and are currently being actively developed. There is now no doubt that large arterial stiffness is a major risk factor for CHD and its pharmacological manipulation presents a novel target for the treatment and prevention of CHD in the future.

This book is intended both as a guide to clinicians interested in the rational treatment of CHD and is written to concentrate particularly on the most frequently asked and important questions and providing, where available, simple, understandable, evidence-based answers. We also hope to appeal to patients concerned about their own health, as we firmly believe that in future the prevention of CHD will depend on greater patient understanding and involvement with the diagnosis, treatment and prevention of this important condition.

DEN
JRC
IBW

Acknowledgements

Special thanks must go to Mrs Janet Usher and Mrs Angela Loveridge for their considerable help to JRC and IBW with preparation of the manuscript.

How to use this book

The *Your Questions Answered* series aims to meet the information needs of GPs and other primary care professionals who care for patients with chronic conditions. It is designed to help them work with patients and their families, providing effective, evidence-based care and management.

The books are in an accessible question and answer format, with detailed contents lists at the beginning of every chapter and a complete index to help find specific information.

ICONS
Icons are used in the book to identify particular types of information:

 highlights information important to clinical practice

 highlights side-effect information.

PATIENT QUESTIONS
At the end of relevant chapters there are sections of frequently asked patient questions, with easy-to-understand answers aimed at the non-medical reader. These questions are also listed at the end of the book.

What is coronary heart disease?

1

1.1 What is coronary heart disease?

Coronary heart disease (CHD) can be defined as relating to disease processes that affect the coronary arterial circulation with consequences for the heart and its function. However, this term is generally restricted to apply only to atherosclerotic coronary artery disease with the consequence of ischaemic heart disease. For the purposes of this book, we will restrict coronary heart disease to this latter specific designation.

1.2 How is coronary heart disease manifested?

Atherosclerotic disease of the coronary arteries (*Fig. 1.1*) can be manifest in many ways. For most individuals, the presence of coronary atheroma is subclinical and asymptomatic. Indeed, ~30% of people aged 20–29 years of age will already have evidence of coronary artery atherosclerosis and this figure exceeds 85% in people aged over 50 years. Thus, most coronary atherosclerotic disease is silent and does not lead to clinical disease.

The two main clinically evident forms of CHD arise from either a fixed chronic obstruction or an acute dynamic occlusion of the coronary artery:

- ■ Angina pectoris (*see Ch. 2*) is the commonest manifestation of CHD and occurs when an atherosclerotic stenosis in the coronary artery impairs the ability of the coronary circulation to increase blood flow

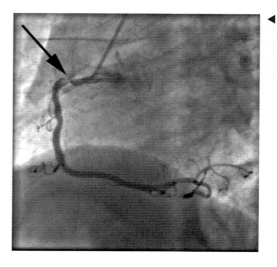

Fig. 1.1 Coronary artery angiogram: right coronary artery with proximal stenosis and in situ thrombus (arrow).

during times of increased cardiac work and myocardial oxygen demand, such as with physiological stress. This is often referred to as a reduced coronary flow reserve and occurs when the luminal stenosis exceeds 70%. This typically causes exercise or stress-induced reversible myocardial ischaemia.

■ The second major manifestation is an acute coronary syndrome (*see Ch. 3*). Here, the coronary atherosclerotic plaque becomes unstable and may rupture. Thrombus deposition over the complex plaque leads to an acute dynamic reduction or cessation in coronary blood flow. This causes myocardial ischaemia at rest that, if transient, is reversible (unstable angina) but will cause irreversible damage with protracted occlusion (myocardial infarction).

For some unfortunate individuals, their first manifestation of CHD is sudden cardiac death. This usually occurs in the context of an acute coronary syndrome and arises due to ischaemia-induced arrhythmic death from ventricular fibrillation.

Myocardial ischaemia may be silent, because of conditions such as degenerative or diabetic autonomic neuropathy, or misinterpreted and ascribed to other conditions, such as indigestion and dyspepsia. This can lead to late clinical presentations with conditions, such as heart failure or recurrent arrhythmias, which arise from the consequences of chronic myocardial ischaemia and infarction.

1.3 What is the incidence and prevalence of coronary heart disease in the UK population?

The British Heart Foundation estimates that the incidence of CHD is up to ~275 000 cases of acute myocardial infarction and ~335 000 cases of angina pectoris per annum in the United Kingdom. However, measures vary and, using Framingham models, more conservative estimates suggest ~250 000 new CHD events per annum including ~125 000 acute myocardial infarctions, ~110 000 cases of angina (stable and unstable) and ~20 000 sudden cardiac deaths.

Although the age-adjusted incidence of CHD has been declining over recent years (~2% per year decline in men), the population prevalence appears to be increasing. This reflects the age-related prevalence of CHD combined with the increasing mean age of the general population: 1–3% of men aged 40–49 have CHD compared with 20–25% of men aged 70–79 years.[1]

1.4 Is the incidence of coronary heart disease similar in all populations and races?

Coronary artery disease is one of the most important causes of premature death in the developed world. The epidemiology of coronary artery disease and angina pectoris is changing. In some regions of the world, such as North America, Western Europe, Japan and Australasia, the age-adjusted incidence, mortality and in-hospital case fatalities are declining, although the overall prevalence of coronary artery disease is still rising in keeping with an ageing population. However, Eastern Europe, in particular, is experiencing escalating rates of coronary artery disease and associated mortality (*Fig. 1.2*).[2]

Coronary atherosclerosis is associated with many risk factors such as cigarette smoking, hyperlipidaemia, family history, hypertension and diabetes mellitus (*see Q. 1.7*). The prevalence and extent of coronary atheroma and angina pectoris increase with age and has a male preponderance. Distribution among ethnic groups is unequal, with higher rates in Indo-Asians and lower rates in East Asians and Afro-Caribbeans in comparison to Caucasians.

1.5 What is the pathophysiology of coronary heart disease?

The predominant underlying cause of CHD is atherosclerosis of the coronary arteries. Atherosclerosis is a chronic process initiated by lipid

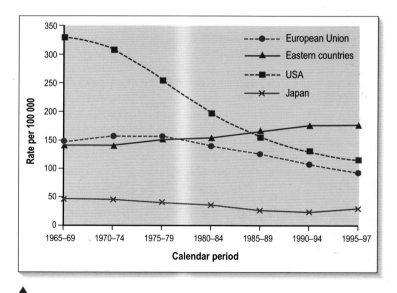

▲

Fig. 1.2 Heart disease across the world. Trends in age-standardised (world population) death certification rates from coronary heart disease in men in all age groups from the European Union, Eastern European countries (Bulgaria, Czech Republic, Hungary, Poland, Romania and Slovakia), the USA and Japan, 1965–1997. (From Levi et al.[2] with permission from the BMJ Publishing Group.)

deposition and vascular wall injury that causes increased endothelial permeability, inflammation and recruitment of monocytes and leucocytes. These latter inflammatory cells accumulate oxidised lipids to form macrophages and foam cells, and lead to the formation of so-called 'fatty streaks'. In an attempt to wall off this inflammatory, lipid-laden deposit, the additional recruitment of vascular smooth muscle cells facilitates the formation of a firm fibrous cap. This fibrotic chronic inflammatory response attempts to contain the necrotic pool of lipids, leucocytes and debris. Further expansion of the atheromatous plaque can occur with continued inflammation and lipid deposition, particularly at the shoulders of the lesion. Such plaque expansion is associated with plaque instability that increases its propensity to rupture and induce coronary thrombosis (*Fig. 1.3*).[3]

Atheromatous encroachment of the vascular lumen causes few symptoms until approximately 70% or more of the luminal area is obstructed. These stenoses do not usually limit coronary blood flow at rest but, with physical exertion, cardiac output rises, leading to an increase in myocardial metabolism and oxygen demands. The coronary resistance

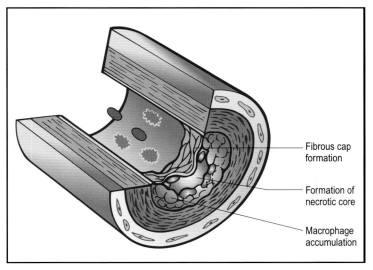

Fibrous cap
formation

Formation of
necrotic core

Macrophage
accumulation

▲

Fig. 1.3 Atherosclerosis is a chronic inflammatory process initiated by lipid deposition and vascular wall injury that causes increased endothelial permeability, inflammation and recruitment of monocytes and leucocytes. (From Newby and Grubb,[3] with permission of Elsevier Ltd.)

vessels dilate in order to increase blood flow to meet these additional requirements. However, the coronary artery stenoses impair the capacity to increase blood flow, resulting in an inability to meet the metabolic demands of the heart. This causes relative myocardial ischaemia and the patient may experience angina pectoris. Relief from angina occurs by either reducing the metabolic demands of the heart, such as by stopping physical exertion, or by causing epicardial coronary vasodilatation, such as with the administration of sublingual nitrates (*see Ch. 6*).

1.6 What are the consequences of a disrupted atheromatous plaque?

The consequences of, and outcomes from, a disrupted atheromatous plaque are potentially three-fold:

1. Acute coronary thrombosis and occlusion (*see Fig. 1.1*) leading to an acute coronary syndrome
2. Plaque growth and expansion causing new onset or deteriorating angina
3. Complete resolution and healing with little or no symptoms (see below).

The ultimate outcome will be determined by a combination of local factors (e.g. plaque structure, inflammation and endothelial function) and systemic variables (e.g. coagulation cascades and platelet activation).

ACUTE CORONARY SYNDROMES

The likelihood of sustaining an acute myocardial infarct increases with the severity and extent of atheromatous involvement of the coronary arteries. In addition, left ventricular function and the frequency of angina, as well as demographics such as age and sex, have an important influence on the risk of myocardial infarction. Most cases of acute myocardial infarction and sudden cardiac death occur in the absence of pre-existing symptoms of angina. This is because, in many cases, thrombus forms on an atheromatous plaque that is not severe enough to limit blood flow. Angiographic studies indicate that in the large majority of cases, the culprit atheromatous plaque that causes acute myocardial infarction encroaches on the luminal diameter by less than 50%. However, coronary angiography may fail to identify, or greatly underestimate the extent of, atheromatous disease. This is because, in the presence of atheroma, the artery may expand to compensate for the plaque and restore the lumen to a normal or near normal size: so-called 'Glagovian remodelling'. This has been widely confirmed by intravascular ultrasound studies and highlights the importance of plaque burden and structure, as opposed to luminal stenosis, when assessing the extent and stability of coronary artery atherosclerosis.

The initiating event of an acute myocardial infarction or sudden cardiac death is often the formation of thrombus on an inflamed atherosclerotic plaque that has eroded or ruptured. Post mortem features associated with plaque rupture and coronary thrombosis include a large lipid-rich core, a thin disorganised collagenous cap and the presence of large numbers of macrophages. Why some plaques cause thrombotic vessel occlusion while adjacent plaques within the same artery remain stable and quiescent is unclear.

ATHEROTHROMBOSIS

Small areas of denudation and thrombus deposition are a common finding on the surface of atheromatous plaques but usually remain subclinical due to endogenous fibrinolysis and 'passification' of the lesion. Detailed post mortem studies have shown that plaque growth is induced by episodic subclinical plaque disruption and thrombus formation. The prolonged presence of residual thrombus over a disrupted or eroded plaque will provoke smooth muscle migration, the production of new connective tissue and consequent plaque expansion.

1.7   What are the risk factors for coronary heart disease?

The propensity to develop, and the subsequent prognosis, of CHD is, in part, determined by a number of risk factors (*see Ch. 5*). The major risk factors are a family history of premature CHD, smoking habit, diabetes mellitus, hypertension and hypercholesterolaemia. A family history of premature CHD is generally accepted to be present when it occurs in a first degree relative below the age of 50 years for a man and 60 years for a woman. It is one of the strongest predictors for the development of CHD.

1.8   What role do lifestyle factors play in coronary heart disease?

Diet plays an important role in modifying the risk for the development of CHD. The high consumption of saturated animal fats (especially those in red meats and dairy products) is associated with an increased risk of CHD. In contrast, a Mediterranean type diet or diets high in omega-3 polyunsaturated fatty acids of fish oils appear to confer a protective and preventative beneficial effect. Modest alcohol consumption is associated with a reduced risk of CHD and should be limited to 21–28 units per week (1 unit = 8 g of absolute alcohol) for a man and 14–21 units per week for a woman. The type of alcoholic beverage is unimportant and undue emphasis has been placed on red wine.

There is a significant and independent association between body mass index and the risk of cardiovascular events. Although an independent risk factor, obesity is also associated with the development of glucose intolerance, frank diabetes mellitus and hypertension. These factors collectively confer an even greater risk.

In comparison to a sedentary lifestyle, regular physical activity is associated with approximately a 50% reduction in the risk of future cardiac events. The benefits appear to relate, in part, to the associated improvements in blood pressure and lipid profile. Most exercise programmes recommend at least 30 minutes of aerobic exercise three times a week. However, there is, paradoxically, an increased risk of sustaining an adverse cardiac event while performing the physical exercise itself. This is clearly offset by the greater benefits accrued following completion of the physical activity. (*See also lifestyle factors in Ch. 5.*)

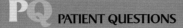

PATIENT QUESTIONS

1.9 What is coronary heart disease?

The heart is a muscle that pumps blood around the body. The coronary arteries are the vessels that supply the heart with blood. A constant blood supply is needed to give the heart all the oxygen and nutrients it needs to keep pumping and beating. Coronary heart disease occurs when these coronary arteries 'fur up' and become blocked by a condition called 'atheroma'. Atheroma is Greek for gruel, reflecting the porridge-like consistency of these fatty deposits that bulge out from the wall of the arteries.

Narrowing of the coronary arteries can have a number of consequences for the heart and for the patient. Coronary heart disease can cause many different symptoms including chest pain, breathlessness, palpitation (heart racing) and tiredness.

Stable angina

2

2.1 What is angina pectoris?

The word 'angina' means choking. Vincent's angina refers to the choking sensation caused by a swollen tongue arising from an infection in the floor of the mouth. Angina pectoris, or 'choking in the chest', is characteristically described as a retrosternal chest discomfort that has a close relation to physical or emotional stress, and is rapidly relieved by rest or nitrates. The chest discomfort is usually described as constricting, pressing or tight, although with so-called 'angina equivalents' it may be manifest by other symptoms, such as breathlessness. Radiation to the arms, jaw, upper abdomen and back may occur either in association or in isolation. In patients with chronic stable angina, the pain is usually initiated at consistent levels of physical stress and promptly disappears with cessation of activity.

2.2 What causes angina pectoris?

Angina pectoris is caused by an imbalance between the metabolic demands of the heart and the myocardial oxygen supply. It is predominantly caused by obstructive coronary atheroma that reduces the capacity of the coronary vasculature to increase blood flow during periods of increased metabolic demand, such as during physical exercise. The induction of myocardial ischaemia during such stress leads to the sensation of angina pectoris although the precise mechanisms and pathways of cardiac neural pain stimulation are incompletely described or understood.

The likelihood that coronary artery disease is the cause of chest pain is increased by the presence of established risk factors, such as smoking and hypertension. There are usually no physical signs in patients with angina but there may be stigmata of hyperlipidaemia (rare) or signs of peripheral vascular disease. All patients should be examined for signs of other causes of angina, such as aortic stenosis and hypertrophic obstructive cardiomyopathy.

2.3 How is the severity of angina classified?

A functional classification has been described by the Canadian Cardiovascular Society (www.ccs.ca) and is the most widely used scale for describing the severity of angina (*Box 2.1*).

2.4 What is the aetiology of angina pectoris?

Obstructive atherosclerotic coronary artery disease is the most common cause, but other cardiac conditions can give rise to anginal pain (*Box 2.2*). Anginal chest pain may also result from an imbalance between myocardial

---

BOX 2.1 The Canadian Cardiovascular Society functional classification of stable angina pectoris

Class 1

Ordinary physical activity, such as walking and climbing stairs, does not cause angina. Angina with strenuous or rapid or prolonged exertion at work or recreation.

Class 2

Slight limitation of ordinary activity. Walking or climbing stairs rapidly, walking uphill, walking or stair climbing after meals, in cold, in wind, or when under emotional stress, or only during the few hours after awakening. Walking more than two blocks on the level and climbing more than one flight of ordinary stairs at a normal pace and in normal conditions.

Class 3

Marked limitation of ordinary physical activity. Walking one to two blocks on the level and climbing more than one flight in normal conditions.

Class 4

Inability to carry on any physical activity without discomfort. Anginal syndrome may be present at rest.

BOX 2.2 The causes of anginal chest pain not attributable to a fixed atheromatous stenosis of the coronary artery

- Vascular disorders
    - variant angina
    - atheroma-associated vasospasm
    - microvascular angina
    - 'Syndrome X'
- Cardiac disorders
    - hypertrophic cardiomyopathy
    - aortic stenosis
    - hypertensive heart disease and left ventricular hypertrophy
    - severe pulmonary hypertension and right ventricular hypertrophy

---

oxygen delivery and the metabolic demands of the heart that is unrelated to coronary blood flow per se – for example, profound anaemia (reduced oxygen delivery) or thyrotoxicosis (increased metabolic demands).

2.5   What is the difference between stable and unstable angina?

By implication, stable angina has a predictable presentation. Anginal symptoms are provoked at a consistent level of physical activity or stress. The provocation of angina may vary with environmental factors, such as cold windy weather, or with the 'warm up' phenomenon where repeated exercise within a short time is better tolerated.

Worsening angina provoked by progressively less exertion over a short period of time, often culminating in pain at rest, is indicative of crescendo angina. New onset angina and crescendo angina are both forms of unstable angina (*see Ch. 3*). Acute unstable angina is characterised by sudden onset of anginal chest pain at rest in the absence of myocardial infarction (*see Q. 3.3*).

2.6   What are the 'angina equivalents'?

Some patients do not describe anginal chest pain when myocardial ischaemia is induced. The most common angina equivalent is dyspnoea although some patients may describe eructation, nausea or indigestion. Such angina equivalents are more common in elderly patients and those with autonomic nervous system dysfunction, such as patients with diabetes mellitus. It should also be recognised that cardiac visceral pain may be referred to the arm or jaw without the development of pain in the chest itself.

2.7   What is the most common form of angina?

The most common form of angina pectoris is characterised by predictable exertional central chest pain that is the consequence of obstructive atheromatous coronary artery disease. Other pathological cardiac conditions can cause angina (*see Box 2.2*), including aortic stenosis and hypertrophic cardiomyopathy. Epicardial vasospasm associated with apparently normal coronary arteries or non-obstructive atheromatous plaques can occur. This can lead to variant or Prinzmetal's angina. The latter rarely gives rise to the typical and predictable exertional chest pain of chronic stable angina.

2.8   What is the prognosis of patients with stable angina?

Angina results in substantial morbidity and mortality. In two-thirds of patients, angina has significant effects on the ability to work, and to undertake recreational, sexual and other daily activities. On average, a patient with angina pectoris will consult a primary health care professional two to three times each year.

The prognosis and complications of angina pectoris relate, in part, to the extent and severity of coronary artery disease and include myocardial infarction, congestive heart failure, arrhythmias and sudden cardiac death.

Risk stratification of patients with angina pectoris is an important process that helps to guide further investigations and management. Simple clinical factors, such as the presence and number of risk factors, previous cardiac history and left ventricular function, can be used to identify those patients who are at particularly high risk. Non-invasive investigations, such as resting electrocardiogram and stress testing, provide important complementary prognostic information and help guide the need for invasive investigation with coronary angiography.

In general, the 5-year mortality rate for patients with stable angina pectoris is 15%. This rises to 25% for those with impaired left ventricular function and to 45% in patients with left main stem stenosis. Patients with mild symptoms, a normal stress test or single vessel disease have a better prognosis.

2.9   What is the risk of developing an acute coronary syndrome?

Overall, patients with stable angina pectoris have a 4–6% risk of death or non-fatal myocardial infarction each year and 30% of those with recent onset angina will have a significant cardiac event (death, non-fatal myocardial infarction or coronary revascularisation) within a year of presentation. However, new onset angina should be classified as a form of unstable angina (*see Ch. 3*) since the precipitant for the development of angina is often plaque rupture and instability.

As with prognosis, the risk of developing an acute coronary syndrome is increased by the extent and severity of the atherosclerotic coronary artery disease. The 5-year risk of sustaining an acute myocardial infarction is 20–25% when the luminal stenosis is greater than 85%. This event rate falls to approximately 10% for intermediate lesions and <3% for stenoses less than 50%. However, for the majority of patients with angina, the stenosis causing the symptoms remains stable and does not inevitably progress to cause an acute coronary syndrome.

PATIENT QUESTIONS

2.10 What is angina?

Angina (or angina pectoris) means a choking sensation in the chest that is caused by 'furring up' of the heart or coronary arteries. Unlike a heart attack, there is no blood clot and the arteries are only partly blocked with enough blood getting through when a person is resting. However, when the heart needs to work harder, such as when climbing a steep hill, it needs more blood to do the extra work. Normally the flow of blood increases to meet the demands of the heart. When the coronary arteries are partly blocked, not enough blood can get through and this causes the heart muscle to struggle. This lack of blood causes a cramping of the heart muscle and the patient feels a pain or discomfort in the chest that is often described as tight or heavy.

The chest pain of angina can spread down the arms, particularly the left arm, or up into the jaw. The pain usually comes on during physical activity and exertion, and is relieved by resting or taking a spray of 'GTN'. Angina does not damage the heart muscle and, in itself, is not life threatening.

Acute coronary syndromes

3

3.1   What is an acute coronary syndrome?

The term 'acute coronary syndrome' encompasses a spectrum of unstable coronary artery disease that includes unstable angina and myocardial infarction. All have a common aetiology in the formation of thrombus on an inflamed and complicated atheromatous plaque. The principles behind the presentation, investigations and management of these syndromes are similar but are subject to important distinctions depending on the category of acute coronary syndrome. The definition of, and distinction between, the acute coronary syndromes relies on the triad of clinical presentation, electrocardiographic changes and biochemical cardiac markers (*Table 3.1*).

3.2   What causes an acute coronary syndrome?

The initiating event of an acute coronary syndrome is the formation of thrombus on an inflamed atherosclerotic plaque that has eroded or ruptured (*see Qs 1.5 and 1.6*). Post mortem findings associated with plaque rupture and coronary thrombosis include a large lipid-rich core, a thin disorganised collagenous cap and the presence of large numbers of inflammatory macrophages.

Secondary causes of acute coronary syndromes result from increases in the metabolic demands of the myocardium or reductions in oxygen delivery to the heart. These usually occur in the presence of obstructive coronary atheroma but without plaque rupture or erosion. Examples include thyrotoxicosis or profound anaemia. Rarely, coronary artery spasm, such as with cocaine abuse, phaeochromocytoma or spontaneous coronary artery dissection, such as with blunt chest trauma, can cause an acute coronary syndrome.

3.3   How are acute coronary syndromes classified?

The main important distinction between classes of acute coronary syndrome relates to the presence or absence of myocardial necrosis since this will determine whether a patient has sustained a myocardial infarction or has unstable angina respectively (*see Table 3.1*).

UNSTABLE ANGINA

Acute unstable angina occurs when a patient has prolonged anginal chest pain at rest in the absence of a precipitant, such as physical or emotional stress. Patients with recent onset angina or angina that is precipitated by progressively less exertion – so-called 'crescendo angina' – also constitute an acute coronary syndrome since it implies plaque growth and instability which is likely to result, in part, from in situ thrombus formation. The Braunwald classification of unstable angina attempts to provide an objective description of the clinical presentation and clinical context as well as the response to therapy (*Box 3.1*).

TABLE 3.1 Classification of acute coronary syndromes

	Clinical presentation	Electrocardiogram	Creatine kinase	Cardiac troponin
Unstable angina				
New onset or crescendo angina	Recent onset or progressively deteriorating established angina	Usually normal. May have ST segment depression or T wave inversion	Normal	Normal
Subacute unstable angina	Stuttering episodes of recurrent angina at rest	ST segment depression, T wave inversion or may be normal	Normal	Normal
Acute unstable angina	Sudden onset of severe anginal chest pain at rest	ST segment depression, T wave inversion or may be normal	Normal	Normal
Myocardial infarction				
Minimal myocardial injury	Sudden onset of severe anginal chest pain at rest	ST segment depression, T wave inversion or may be normal	Normal	Elevated
Acute sub-endocardial myocardial infarction	Sudden onset of severe anginal chest pain at rest	ST segment elevation or depression, bundle branch block, T wave inversion or may be normal. No new Q waves	Elevated	Elevated
Acute transmural myocardial infarction	Sudden onset of severe anginal chest pain at rest	ST segment elevation, bundle branch block, T wave inversion, Q waves	Elevated	Elevated

MYOCARDIAL INFARCTION

Myocardial infarction occurs when there is pathological or biochemical evidence of myocyte necrosis (*Box 3.2*). This may be classified in several different ways but is usually categorised according to the clinical features of the electrocardiogram: territory, ST segment shifts or Q waves. The most important classification relates to the presence of ST segment elevation or bundle branch block since this determines the immediate management of the patient (*see Ch. 9*). The territory and development of Q waves provide

---

BOX 3.1   Braunwald classification of unstable angina

Clinical presentation

■ Class I: New onset, severe or accelerated angina
  — *Patients with angina of less than 2 months' duration, severe or occurring three or more times per day, or angina that is distinctly more frequent and precipitated by distinctly less exertion. No rest pain in the last 2 months.*

■ Class II: Angina at rest – subacute
  — *Patients with one or more episodes of angina at rest during the preceding month but not within the preceding 48 hours.*

■ Class III: Angina at rest – acute
  — *Patients with one or more episodes of angina at rest during the preceding 48 hours.*

Clinical context

■ Class A: Secondary unstable angina
  — *A clearly defined condition extrinsic to the coronary vascular bed that has intensified myocardial ischaemia, e.g. anaemia, infection, fever, hypotension, tachyarrhythmia, thyrotoxicosis, hypoxaemia.*

■ Class B: Primary unstable angina

■ Class C: Post myocardial infarction unstable angina
  — *Within 2 weeks of documented myocardial infarction.*

Therapeutic intervention

■ Absence of, or minimal treatment.

■ Occurring in the presence of standard therapy for chronic stable angina.

■ Occurring despite maximally tolerated doses of all three categories of oral therapy, including intravenous nitrates.

Class IIIB has been further subdivided into IIIB-T_{pos} and IIIB-T_{neg} to reflect the marked differences in prognostic risk conferred by the presence or absence of an elevation in troponin I or T concentrations. NB: This ignores the WHO classification of myocardial infarction that includes an elevation in the troponin concentration.

---

important prognostic information: patients with anterior Q wave infarction have a poorer prognosis.

3.4   What are cardiac troponins and how are they used?

Cardiac enzymes and markers are the principal determinants that define the category of the acute coronary syndrome. Creatine kinase, aspartate transferase and lactate dehydrogenase are the 'classic' cardiac enzymes that are measured to confirm the presence or absence of myocardial necrosis (*see*

BOX 3.2 Definitions of myocardial infarction

Original WHO definition

A combination of two of three characteristics:

1. Typical symptoms (i.e. chest discomfort)
2. Cardiac enzyme rise ($\geq$ twice the upper limit of the normal reference range)
3. Typical electrocardiogram (ECG) pattern involving the development of Q waves.

ESC/ACC definition of myocardial infarction

Criteria for acute, evolving or recent MI

Either one of the following criteria satisfies the diagnosis for an acute, evolving or recent MI:

1. Typical rise and gradual fall (troponin) or more rapid rise and fall (creatine kinase MB isoenzyme (CK-MB)) of biochemical markers of myocardial necrosis with at least one of the following:
   a. ischaemic symptoms
   b. development of pathologic Q waves on the ECG
   c. ECG changes indicative of ischaemia (ST segment elevation or depression)
   d. coronary artery intervention (e.g. coronary angioplasty).
2. Pathologic findings of an acute MI.

Criteria for established MI

Either one of the following criteria satisfies the diagnosis for established MI:

1. Development of new pathologic Q waves on serial ECGs. The patient may or may not remember previous symptoms. Biochemical markers of myocardial necrosis may have normalised, depending on the length of time that has passed since the infarct developed.
2. Pathologic findings of a healed or healing MI.

Biochemical markers

The following are biochemical indicators for detecting myocardial necrosis:

1. Maximal concentration of troponin T or I exceeding the decision limit (99th percentile of the values for a reference control group) on at least one occasion during the first 24 hours after the index clinical event.
2. Maximal value of CK-MB (preferably CK-MB mass) exceeding the 99th percentile of the values for a reference control group on two successive samples, or maximal value exceeding twice the upper limit of normal for the specific institution on one occasion during the first hours after the index clinical event.

BOX 3.2 Definitions of myocardial infarction—cont'd

Values for CK-MB should rise and fall; values that remain elevated without change are almost never due to MI. In the absence of availability of a troponin or CK-MB assay, total CK (greater than two times the upper reference limit) or the B fraction of CK may be employed, but these last two biomarkers are considerably less satisfactory than CK-MB.

Box 3.2). They have a characteristic release profile with creatine kinase peaking first at around 12 hours (*Fig. 3.1*). These three enzymes are not specific to the heart but can also be released by such disparate tissues as skeletal muscle, liver and erythrocytes. However, different tissues express the various isoforms of each enzyme to a varying degree. For example, the MB isoform of creatine kinase is expressed at higher levels in the heart and can be used to discriminate cardiac injury from the release of creatine kinase from other tissues.

Recently, there has been a major advance in the assessment of myocardial damage through the measurement of the cardiac markers, troponin I and troponin T. These structural proteins and cofactors are involved in the binding of calcium during myocyte contraction and are highly specific to the myocardium. They are released from the myocardium following tissue necrosis, with peak plasma concentrations being detected at 10–12 hours although they may be elevated within 6 hours. The plasma concentrations may remain elevated for 7 days, or longer in the presence of renal impairment. Estimations of cardiac troponins are particularly useful in the management of patients with chest pain of uncertain aetiology.

The cardiac troponins are extremely sensitive to myocardial injury and damage, such that very small amounts of damage can be detected. This has meant that 'micro-infarcts' can be detected where there is an elevation in the troponin concentration without a significant rise in the creatine kinase or other cardiac enzymes. Because of this, confusion has arisen in the distinction between unstable angina and myocardial infarction. During the widespread introduction of troponin measurements, a patient presenting with an acute coronary syndrome who had a normal creatine kinase and an elevated troponin would be classified as having unstable angina. Subsequently, the European Society of Cardiology (ESC) and the American College of Cardiology (ACC) ruled that any elevation in a cardiac marker or enzyme should be taken as evidence of myocardial necrosis and that the patient should be classified as having had a myocardial infarct, however small. This has led some clinicians to classify such patients as having 'minimal myocardial injury' (*see Table 3.1*).

The measurement of cardiac markers and enzymes in the first 24 hours provides not only diagnostic but also prognostic information in patients with an acute coronary syndrome. As with the electrocardiogram, an elevation in the cardiac troponin identifies those patients who are at greatest risk (*Fig. 3.2*) and who would benefit from more aggressive therapeutic intervention.[1]

The high degree of sensitivity associated with cardiac troponins is associated with some problems in interpretation. Troponin release may also

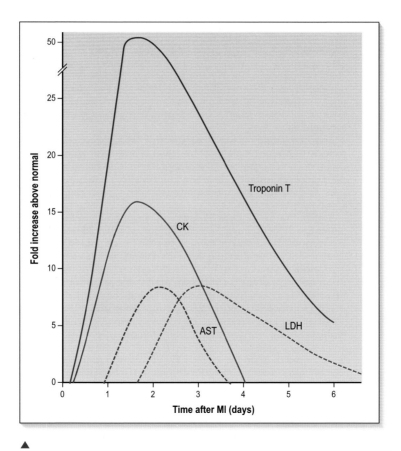

Fig. 3.1 Profile of cardiac enzymes following an acute myocardial infarction. AST, aspartate transferase; CK, creatine kinase; LDH, lactate dehydrogenase.

occur in other contexts where the heart is under stress, such as pulmonary thromboembolism, cardiomyopathies and supraventricular tachycardias. Whilst a rise in cardiac troponin is specific to the heart, it is not necessarily specific to acute coronary syndromes.

3.5 What role does the electrocardiogram have in the diagnosis of acute coronary syndromes?

The electrocardiogram will often show evidence of ischaemia that classically takes the form of ST segment shifts, T wave inversion and new bundle branch block (*Fig. 3.3*). However, it is not uncommon for the electrocardiogram to appear normal, particularly at first presentation. It is important to undertake repeated electrocardiograms, especially in the presence of persisting ongoing chest pain, because the electrocardiogram often evolves and develops new ischaemic changes. Indeed, a patient may rapidly progress from unstable angina and an apparently normal electrocardiogram to an acute transmural myocardial infarct with ST segment elevation.

In unstable angina, ischaemic electrocardiographic changes provide important markers of an adverse prognosis with the presence, and degree, of ST segment depression being independent predictors of mortality. They also identify those patients with the most to gain from therapeutic interventions such as percutaneous coronary intervention.

Bundle branch block or ST segment elevation identifies those patients with acute myocardial infarction who would benefit from intravenous thrombolytic therapy or primary angioplasty. Although ST segment depression may occur in patients with an acute myocardial infarction (especially in the posterior territory), thrombolytic therapy is contraindicated in these cases because such treatment is associated with a higher overall mortality.

The electrocardiogram provides information about the territory of ischaemia and even the affected coronary artery. Inferior ischaemia is represented by electrocardiographic changes in leads II, III and aVF, and usually relates to the right coronary artery. Anterior ischaemia is represented by changes in leads V2–V6, relating to the left anterior descending coronary artery. Posterolateral ischaemia is represented by leads I, aVL, V6 and 'reciprocal' changes in V2–V4, relating to the circumflex artery. The relative contribution of the circumflex and right coronary arteries to inferior and lateral myocardial perfusion is quite variable.

The development of new Q waves indicates the presence of transmural infarction. This suggests more extensive myocardial damage than non-Q wave myocardial infarction, although this may be misleading.

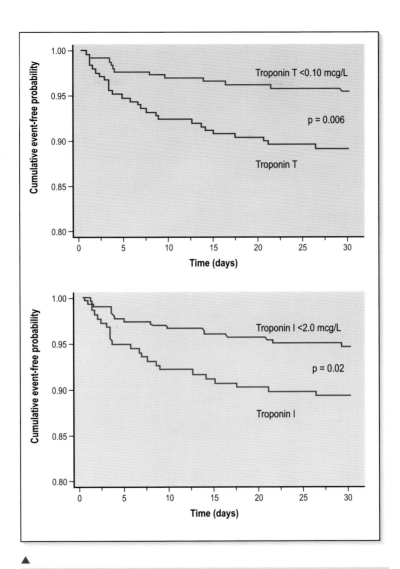

Fig. 3.2 Predictive value of troponin I and troponin T in patients with acute coronary syndrome. (From Luscher et al.[1] with permission).

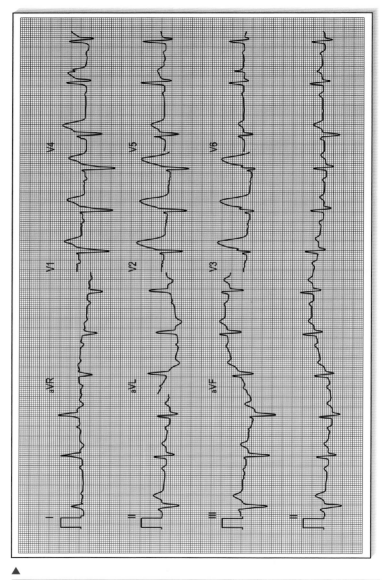

Fig. 3.3 An ECG from a patient with an acute anterior myocardial infarction. Note the large T waves and ST segment elevation in the anterior chest leads (V1–V5).

3.6 How is unstable angina distinguished from myocardial infarction?

The distinction between unstable angina and myocardial infarction has recently undergone significant change. Previously, unstable angina referred to patients who had not fulfilled the WHO criteria for myocardial infarction but had anginal chest pain with or without ischaemic electrocardiographic changes. With the advent of cardiac troponin estimations, many patients with normal or marginal creatinine kinase rises could be identified as having cardiac chest pain and were termed 'troponin positive unstable angina' (*see Box 3.1*). However, from basic principles, this does not make sense since myocyte necrosis is necessary to induce troponin release and this was the rationale for the joint statement from the European Society of Cardiology and the American College of Cardiology (*see Box 3.2*). This new definition of myocardial infarction, in some ways, simplifies the categorisation of acute coronary syndromes. Thus, the distinction between myocardial infarction and unstable angina relies entirely on the presence or absence of a rise in a cardiac marker or enzyme (*see Box 3.1*).

3.7 What are the prognostic markers in patients with an acute coronary syndrome?

Patients with an acute coronary syndrome generally have a poor prognosis. There are several simple clinical markers that identify those patients who are at particularly high risk. Crudely, the number of cardiovascular risk factors is proportional to the future risk. Age is one of the strongest markers of risk. The in-hospital mortality from acute myocardial infarction is ~5% for a 40–50 year old man rising to more than 30% when over 75 years of age. Other adverse clinical factors include left ventricular impairment, renal failure, other vascular disease, diabetes mellitus, delayed (not within the first 48 hours) ventricular arrhythmias, and pulmonary oedema or haemodynamic compromise at presentation.

An increasing number of biochemical markers have been associated with an increased risk. These include peak troponin, C-reactive protein and cholesterol concentrations. However, the electrocardiogram remains one of the strongest independent predictors of risk.

3.8 How can the future risk for patients with acute coronary syndrome be calculated?

There have been several attempts to develop simple clinically applicable scoring systems that can usefully predict the future risk of patients with acute coronary syndromes. The thrombolysis in myocardial infarction (TIMI) risk score was developed from patients who participated in randomised controlled trials of low molecular weight heparin for acute coronary syndromes. This scoring system is simple and easy to apply and relies on the following seven elements:

- Age ≥65 years
- Three or more risk factors for coronary artery disease
- Significant coronary stenosis
- ST segment deviation
- Severe anginal symptoms (two or more anginal events in last 24 hours)
- Prior aspirin use (within last 7 days)
- Elevated serum cardiac markers

These elements are equally weighted to generate a 14-day event rate (*Table 3.2*).

There is a concern that risk scores derived from carefully selected patient populations that are recruited to randomised controlled trials may not be applicable to the normal range of patients encountered in clinical practice. The Global Registry of Acute Coronary Events (GRACE) is more comprehensive and is derived from a registry of unselected patient populations hospitalised with acute coronary syndromes (*see Table 8.1*). Although there is some broad agreement with the TIMI risk score, other factors have also been identified as being highly predictive of outcome, such as renal function, hypotension and the presence of pre-hospital cardiac arrest.

TABLE 3.2 TIMI risk score: 14-day event rate

	Number of risk factors	**14-day event rate**
Low risk	0/1	4.7
	2	8.3
Medium risk	3	13.2
	4	19.9
High risk	5	26.2
	6/7	40.9

PQ PATIENT QUESTIONS

3.9   What is a myocardial infarction?

A myocardial infarction (or MI) occurs when there is a sudden and complete loss of blood supply to a region of the heart. This usually occurs when a blood clot forms on a deposit of atheroma (*see Q. 3.2*) and it completely blocks the artery. This means that the heart muscle supplied by this blocked artery receives no blood and the muscle dies. This is often called a 'heart attack'. The heart muscle then forms a scar. How well the heart performs after a heart attack depends upon how much muscle is damaged and how much of a scar forms.

When a patient suffers a heart attack or 'MI', they often describe a severe pain or heaviness in the chest, associated with sweatiness, sickness and shortness of breath. Nothing seems to get rid of the pain which continues until treatment is given. It is a serious life-threatening condition and patients must seek urgent medical attention.

Clinical assessment in patients with CHD

4

4.1 What are the symptoms of CHD?

The dominant symptom of coronary heart disease (CHD) is chest pain. Typical cardiac ischaemic pain is described as a 'heaviness', 'tightness' or 'constriction' in the chest that radiates to the left arm or jaw. With reversible ischaemia of chronic stable angina, this chest pain is predictable, exertional and of short duration (<20 min) with rapid relief with rest or the administration of short-acting nitrate preparations (see Q. 2.1). Prolonged cardiac chest pain at rest suggests an acute coronary syndrome (see Ch. 3), especially when associated with autonomic symptoms such as sweating. Patients with an acute coronary syndrome may present on a background of chronic stable angina or as a de novo phenomenon. The length of time, the severity of discomfort or pain and the presence of autonomic symptoms (sweating, palor, nausea, breathlessness) are markers of the magnitude of the ischaemic insult. Patients with persistent chest pain lasting more than 20 minutes should seek urgent medical attention because of the likelihood of myocardial damage and infarction.

Other symptoms of CHD usually reflect secondary complications. Breathlessness and fatigue suggest the development of left ventricular dysfunction and heart failure. Palpitation may indicate the development of atrial or ventricular arrhythmias arising from myocardial scar tissue or left ventricular impairment. However, some symptoms may represent 'angina equivalent' (see Q. 2.6) and the clinician should be alert to this possibility. Occasionally, syncope may occur due to ischaemia induced bradyarrhythmias or ventricular tachyarrhythmias.

HISTORY AND EXAMINATION

4.2 Is this cardiac or non-cardiac chest pain?

A careful record of symptoms is essential. For stable anginal pain, the most discerning symptoms are the predictable relationship of the chest pain to exertion and stress, and the radiation of this pain to the neck or jaw. Relief with glyceryl trinitrate is often cited as evidence of myocardial ischaemia but this is neither very specific nor discriminatory, with relief apparent in many cases of non-ischaemic chest pain.

4.3 What are the clinical risk factors?

The likelihood of CHD is increased in the presence of risk factors. The number and nature of risk factors can usefully inform the level of suspicion and indication for onward referral or investigation. Risk prediction charts for primary prevention can assist in the assessment of the likelihood of CHD. However, an over-riding consideration is a prior history of CHD and its severity.

It is also important to enquire about atherosclerosis affecting other areas of the body, such as cerebrovascular and peripheral vascular disease. Patients with a history of these atheroscleroses per se are more likely to die from CHD than through a stroke or ruptured aortic aneurysm.

4.4   How are stability and severity of symptoms assessed?

An essential aspect of the history is the stability of the CHD. Protracted chest pain at rest (>20 min), unrelieved by repeated (×3) sublingual nitrates and associated autonomic symptoms (nausea, sweating, breathlessness) suggest an acute coronary syndrome which mandates emergency admission to hospital.

Patients with new onset angina or crescendo angina represent a high-risk group and should be considered for urgent specialist referral and assessment within 1–2 weeks. Where pain deteriorates, such that it is occurring at rest, the patient should be promptly admitted to hospital.

Patients with severe symptoms, impaired left ventricular function, malignant arrhythmias or poor exercise tolerance have a worse prognosis.

4.5   What are the key points to look for on examination?

There are no typical physical signs in patients with CHD. General examination may, however, reveal stigmata of hyperlipidaemia (rare), tobacco use (nicotine-stained fingers), hypertension, diabetes mellitus (glycosuria) or signs of peripheral and cerebrovascular disease, such as aortic aneurysms and carotid bruits. Other physical signs relate to the complications of CHD, such as signs of left ventricular failure including raised jugular venous pressure, peripheral oedema and chest crepitations. Examination should also include a search for signs of conditions that exacerbate the symptoms of CHD, such as anaemia and thyrotoxicosis, as well as those conditions that may be confused with CHD, such as aortic stenosis and hypertrophic obstructive cardiomyopathy.

INVESTIGATIONS

4.6   What laboratory investigations are required?

In patients with suspected CHD, all patients should have a generalised clinical biochemical and haematological screen. This permits the assessment of risk factors for CHD including hyperlipidaemia (lipid profile), diabetes mellitus (random blood glucose), and renal failure and hypertension (urea, creatinine and electrolytes). Secondary causes or exacerbating factors, such as thyrotoxicosis (thyroid function) and anaemia (full blood count), should be assessed. Where statin therapy is being contemplated, baseline liver function should be documented.

4.7   Should inflammatory markers be measured?

Atherosclerosis is an inflammatory disease process with cycles of vascular damage causing plaque expansion and disruption that may lead to angina, crescendo angina and acute coronary syndromes. Recent epidemiological and observational studies have suggested a link between systemic inflammation and coronary artery disease.[1,2] Markers of systemic inflammation, such as C-reactive protein, serum amyloid A, interleukin-6 and tumour necrosis factor α, are elevated in patients with cardiovascular disease and are associated with adverse prognosis and recurrent coronary events (*Fig. 4.1*). Moreover, in previously healthy individuals, elevated plasma concentrations of C-reactive protein and interleukin-6 have been shown to predict the development of cardiovascular disease (*Fig. 4.2*).

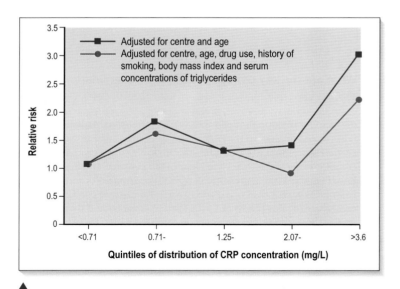

Fig. 4.1 Relative risk of coronary events by quintiles of distribution of CRP concentration in patients with angina. (From Haverkate et al.[1] Reprinted with permission from Elsevier.)

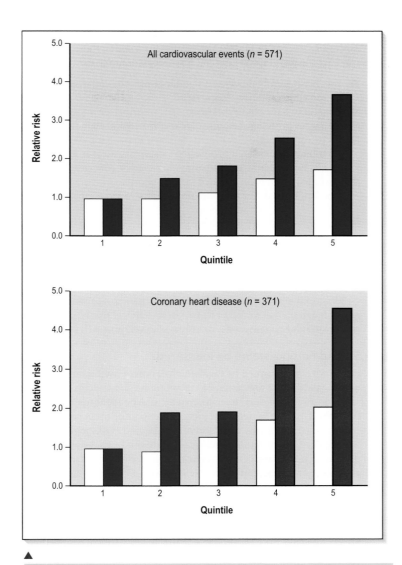

Fig. 4.2 The relationship between CRP and LDL-cholesterol levels and cardiovascular risk in apparently healthy women. Age-adjusted relative risk of future cardiovascular events, according to base-line C-reactive protein levels (solid bars) and LDL cholesterol levels (open bars). (From Ridker et al.[2] Copyright © 2002 Massachusetts Medical Society. All rights reserved.)

Markers of inflammation provide a further novel measure of future cardiovascular risk in both healthy individuals and in those with established vascular disease. However, several issues remain unresolved:

- There is currently no clinical standard or international reference range for these inflammatory markers.
- The additive benefit of this prognostic information above established risk factor profiling remains to be confirmed and validated.
- There are no specific treatments targeted at reducing systemic inflammation although established treatments, such as aspirin and statins, do reduce serum inflammatory marker concentrations.
- Documentation of an elevated inflammatory marker may identify those at additional risk but this does not alter management beyond established therapies, such as statin therapy.
- The reproducibility of these measurements needs to be documented. Measurements of inflammatory markers to assess the future risk of cardiovascular events are invalid when patients have a systemic inflammatory condition, such as an acute respiratory infection or rheumatoid arthritis.

Measurement of systemic inflammatory markers is at an early stage of research and has yet to define its role in the clinical management or risk stratification of patients with, or at risk of developing, CHD.

4.8 Should homocysteine be measured?

Homocysteine is formed by the demethylation of methionine and is an intermediate in the formation of cystathionine and cysteine. The trans-sulphuration of homocysteine to cysteine is dependent upon pyridoxine (vitamin B_6), and the demethylation of methionine upon cobalamin (vitamin B_{12}) and folate. Ingestion of large amounts of methionine, such as with chicken consumption, produces a transient but substantial elevation in plasma homocysteine concentrations. Conversely, pyridoxine, cobalamin and folate supplementation is associated with a reduction in elevated fasting homocysteine concentrations.

Elevated plasma homocysteine concentrations are associated with the development of premature coronary artery disease.[3] This observation has generated a lot of interest since hyperhomocysteinaemia may represent a novel risk factor for CHD that is potentially amenable to simple therapeutic intervention with folate, pyridoxine and cobalamin supplementation. However, there is currently no definitive evidence that such vitamin interventions have any clinically meaningful secondary preventative benefits. The effectiveness of such supplementation in reducing plasma homocysteine concentrations is modest (~10–15% reduction). In rare cases of patients with homozygous methylene tetrahydrofolate reductase deficiency, plasma homocysteine concentrations are much higher, the association with CHD stronger and the reductions with folate supplementation more substantial. However, the clinical benefits of such therapy still remain unproven, albeit theoretically promising.

Currently, there is little evidence that systematically screening plasma homocysteine concentrations in all patients with CHD is worthwhile or helpful.

4.9 Do all patients need an electrocardiogram?

A resting electrocardiogram (ECG) should always be recorded in patients with, or suspected of having, CHD. The ECG can provide both diagnostic and prognostic information.

Changes of a previous transmural myocardial infarction (presence of pathological Q waves) may confirm the diagnosis of coronary artery disease. ST segment and T wave changes also strongly suggest underlying coronary artery disease. However, the resting ECG is not a sensitive test for the diagnosis of coronary artery disease as it is normal in more than 50% of patients presenting with angina but it does provide prognostic information (*Table 4.1*). Resting ST segment depression predicts an increased likelihood of subsequent myocardial infarction and death. Patients with evidence of previous myocardial infarction or ST–T wave abnormalities without transmural Q wave infarction have a reduced survival. Left ventricular hypertrophy is associated with aortic stenosis, hypertrophic cardiomyopathy and hypertension (*Fig. 4.3*).

4.10 Who needs a chest x-ray?

A chest x-ray provides limited information in patients with CHD. It has no role in the diagnosis of coronary atheroma per se, but can identify the presence of complications arising from CHD, such as heart failure, or provide evidence to support alternative diagnoses, such as mediastinal widening in aortic dissection – an important differential diagnosis in

TABLE 4.1 Risk stratification with resting electrocardiogram		
Low risk	**Medium risk**	**High risk**
Normal	ST segment depression ≤1 mm	ST segment elevation
T wave flattening	T wave inversion >1 mm	ST segment depression >1 mm
T wave inversion <1 mm		Deep symmetrical T wave inversion

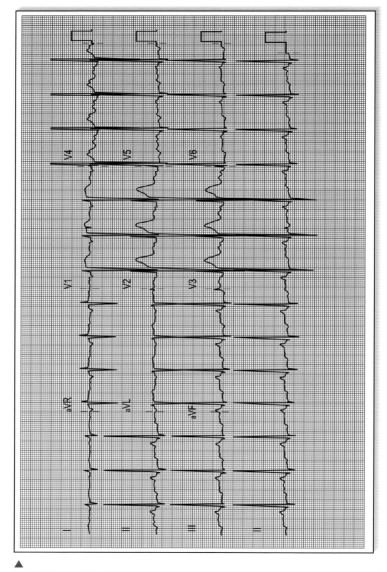

▲

Fig. 4.3 Marked left ventricular hypertrophy due to malignant hypertension.

patients presenting with sudden onset of severe chest pain. The cardiothoracic ratio is a relatively poor way of identifying patients with left ventricular dysfunction and dilatation. An increased cardiothoracic ratio has very poor sensitivity and low specificity for the detection of heart failure. However, it is very useful for the detection of pulmonary oedema and pleural effusions.

A chest x-ray is not routinely appropriate for all patients with CHD. It should be considered in those patients with prominent symptoms of breathlessness or where alternative diagnoses are under consideration.

4.11 Do all patients need an echocardiogram?

Few patients with CHD need an echocardiogram. The diagnosis of CHD may be inferred from the resting echocardiogram such as the presence of a regional wall motion abnormality indicating prior myocardial infarction. However, many patients with CHD will have normal left ventricular function and a normal resting echocardiogram. Stress echocardiography (*see Q. 4.18*) can be used to diagnose CHD but this is technically challenging, not widely available and highly observer dependent. The main diagnostic utility of echocardiography is to confirm alternative diagnoses of cardiac chest pain such as aortic stenosis or hypertrophic obstructive cardiomyopathy.

In patients with suspected complications of CHD, echocardiography should be considered when assessing cardiac performance, such as left ventricular and valvular function. This helps to identify those patients who may benefit from specific therapy such as angiotensin converting enzyme inhibition (*see Ch. 10*).

Left ventricular systolic dysfunction is the most common complication associated with CHD. However, it is very unusual in the presence of a normal resting electrocardiogram and the latter may be used to determine if a breathless patient with suspected CHD should undergo echocardiography.

4.12 Should lipids be assessed only in the fasting state?

Serum cholesterol concentrations are unaffected by acute food ingestion. However, a fasting blood sample may be necessary to obtain a full lipid profile.

Most laboratories currently measure serum total cholesterol, high-density lipoprotein (HDL) cholesterol and triglyceride concentrations. The low-density lipoprotein (LDL) cholesterol concentration is back calculated from these three variables using the Friedewald formula. Unlike cholesterol concentrations, triglyceride concentrations are heavily dependent upon recent food ingestion, especially fatty foods. Thus, using this indirect method, estimation of LDL cholesterol concentrations cannot be made in the non-fasted state.

Primary prevention guidelines use the ratio of total and high-density lipoprotein cholesterol concentrations and therefore do not require a fasting blood sample. Secondary prevention guidelines usually rely upon measurements of total cholesterol concentrations and again do not require a fasting blood sample. However, specific measurement of LDL cholesterol concentrations is occasionally required and, where indirect measurements are made, a fasting blood sample is necessary. Clearly, this also applies to patients with mixed hyperlipidaemias where the fasting triglyceride concentrations are elevated.

REFERRAL TO SECONDARY CARE

4.13 Who should be referred to a cardiologist?

The diagnosis of CHD has many social, psychological and clinical implications for an affected individual. Accurate diagnosis and risk stratification are essential, and onward referral for a cardiology opinion should be considered in all patients. Rapid access chest pain clinics help to provide ready access to a cardiology assessment and opinion. This potentially avoids unnecessary hospitalisation as well as improving the detection of patients with CHD. The criteria for referral vary widely and are dictated by local service provision.

In general, there are three main reasons for onward referral for a specialist cardiology opinion:

1. Confirmation of the diagnosis may be necessary, especially in patients with atypical or unclear symptoms.
2. It is important to risk stratify patients with CHD to guide future investigations and management, such as coronary angiography and coronary revascularisation.
3. Specialist input is often invaluable to ensure the appropriate initiation of anti-anginal and secondary preventative therapies as well as to treat secondary complications such as heart failure.

STRESS TESTING

4.14 Who needs an exercise tolerance test?

Stress testing is performed for two main reasons: to diagnose ischaemic heart disease and to assess prognosis. Occasionally, it may be undertaken to assess cardiac arrhythmias or to evaluate patients who are under consideration for cardiac transplantation. The method of testing can be categorised in two ways:

■ the type of stress: exercise or pharmacological stress (*see Q. 4.15*)
■ the type of test: electrocardiography (*see Q. 4.16*), radionuclide

scintigraphy, echocardiography (*see Q. 4.18*), and occasionally ventilatory gas exchange.

The selection of the most appropriate stress test depends, to a large extent, upon the characteristics of the patient and the indication for the test.

Stress testing is contraindicated in certain high-risk patient groups including patients with severe aortic stenosis, uncontrolled hypertension or acute coronary syndromes. Conversely, it may be required in asymptomatic individuals, such as heavy goods or public service vehicle drivers, with known or suspected coronary artery disease (*see Q. 4.16*).

Treadmill exercise electrocardiography is the commenest form of stress testing. The two other main forms of stress testing are stress myocardial perfusion scintigraphy and stress echocardiography. They are used less frequently than treadmill exercise electrocardiography but can provide additional or complementary information (*see Qs 4.17 and 4.18*).

4.15 What is exertional and pharmacological stress testing?

EXERTIONAL STRESS

Although cycle ergometers offer some advantages, treadmills are the most common method of performing exercise testing. This is because most patients are not experienced cyclists and fatigue of the quadriceps muscles can prematurely limit their activity. The standard treadmill exercise test is the Bruce Protocol where the patient walks on a motorized treadmill and the speed and elevation increase every 3 minutes (*Table 4.2*). A modified Bruce Protocol would be appropriate for patients with poor mobility and is sometimes considered in patients with a potential unstable condition such as suspected unstable angina.

PHARMACOLOGICAL STRESS

Exercise testing in patients with limited mobility is sometimes not feasible. Moreover, for some modalities of assessment, such as stress echocardiography, motion of the patient significantly hinders data interpretation. Under such circumstances, pharmacological stress, with

TABLE 4.2 The Bruce Protocol

	Speed	Elevation	METS	Time
Stage 1	1.7	10%	5	3 min
Stage 2	2.5	12%	7	3 min
Stage 3	3.4	14%	10	3 min
Stage 4	4.2	16%	13	3 min

METS, metabolic equivalents.

intravenous infusions of dobutamine and dipyridamole, is often utilised to cause a rise in cardiac work and oxygen demand by producing a tachycardia, systemic vasodilatation and a high cardiac output.

4.16 How is exercise electrocardiography performed?

The most common and simplest form of stress testing is the treadmill exercise electrocardiogram (*Fig. 4.4*).

BASIC PRINCIPLES

Exercise electrocardiography involves the continuous recording of a standard 12-lead electrocardiogram during a defined level of physical exertional stress. The features of exercise electrocardiography that are most informative include changes in the ST segments (depression or elevation), the blood pressure, ventricular arrhythmias and the patient's symptoms. Depression of the ST segment is the most common sign of myocardial ischaemia on the stress electrocardiogram but the morphology of the ST segment change is crucial with up-sloping ST segment changes unlikely to

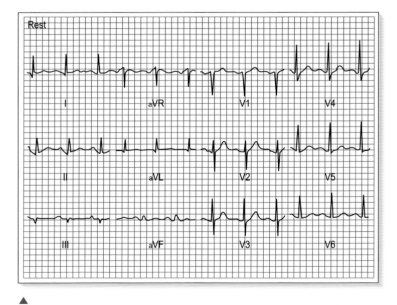

▲

Fig. 4.4 Stress ECG testing. **A,** A normal resting electrocardiogram in a patient with angina.

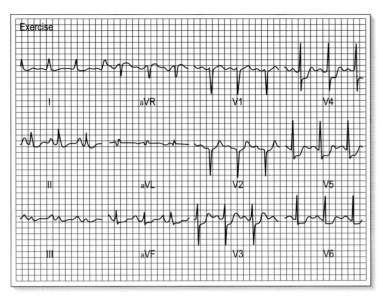

Fig. 4.4 Stress ECG testing. **B**, On exercise there is both horizontal and downsloping ST-segment depression in the anterior chest leads associated with the development of chest pain.

indicate significant myocardial ischaemia. The specificity and sensitivity of the test are improved if the patient is able to achieve 85% of their target heart rate (220 – age for a man; 210 – age for a woman) during exercise.

CLINICAL APPLICATION

Exercise electrocardiography is an inappropriate screening test for ischaemic heart disease when used in isolation. In a population with a low prevalence of ischaemic heart disease, the false positive rate is high, particularly in asymptomatic younger individuals and women.

The clinical context, associated symptoms and overall cardiovascular response to exercise can be as important as the electrocardiographic response to exercise itself. When used appropriately, exercise testing is a reliable, easily performed and robust method of risk stratification in patients with coronary heart disease. It is a particularly useful method of identifying those individuals at highest risk and those who would benefit from further and potentially more invasive investigation and intervention, such as coronary angiography and revascularisation.

The Driver and Vehicle Licensing Agency stipulates that drivers wishing to hold a group II (heavy goods or public service vehicle) licence must conform to certain prespecified regulations if they have known or suspected coronary artery disease. In order to retain a group II licence, patients must be free of anginal symptoms and be able to complete stage 3 of the Bruce Protocol (*see Table 4.2*), without anginal symptoms or ischaemic changes on the electrocardiogram, having been withdrawn from anti-anginal therapy for more than 48 hours.

4.17 What is stress myocardial perfusion scintigraphy?

BASIC PRINCIPLES

This technique uses the principle that myocardial perfusion will dictate the relative myocardial uptake of an intravenously injected radionuclide tracer. During stress (exercise or pharmacological), myocardial uptake will be reduced distal to a significant coronary stenosis in comparison to adjacent territories with normal perfusion. This differential effect will be lost following a period of rest and redistribution unless the area of myocardium has undergone infarction.

To perform stress myocardial perfusion scintigraphy, the patient is injected with the radionuclide tracer at the height of exertional or pharmacological stress. The γ-emissions are then recorded by a γ-camera immediately after the stress and following a period of sustained rest: from 4 hours to the following day depending on the type of tracer (*Fig. 4.5*).

CLINICAL APPLICATION

Stress myocardial perfusion imaging or scintigraphy is a more accurate method of diagnosing ischaemic heart disease than exercise electrocardiography: sensitivity of 80% versus 70%, and specificity of 90% versus 80%, respectively. However, stress myocardial scintigraphy adds little additional information in those patients already identified as high risk using conventional exercise testing. It is particularly helpful in those individuals who have equivocal exercise electrocardiographic changes, an abnormal resting electrocardiogram, suspected false positive or negative exercise electrocardiograms, or submaximal exercise tolerance. It may also prove useful in identifying the territory of ischaemia in patients with multivessel disease where selective revascularisation strategies, such as culprit lesion angioplasty, are being considered. Finally, identification of so-called 'hibernating' myocardium may be of particular benefit in patients with left ventricular dysfunction who have the most to gain from coronary revascularisation.

Short axis

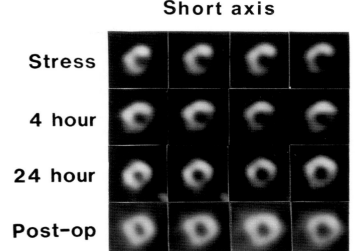

Stress

4 hour

24 hour

Post-op

▲

Fig. 4.5 Myocardial perfusion scintigraphy. Stress, 4-hour, 24-hour and postoperative short-axis thallium-201 myocardial perfusion tomograms in a patient with stable angina. Stress images demonstrated perfusion defects in the lateral wall of the left ventricle which persisted in the 4-hour redistribution images. Redistribution images at 24 hours, however, revealed almost normal uptake of the same regions, indicating the presence of viable ischaemic myocardium. Following successful coronary artery bypass surgery, normal perfusion of the left ventricular wall is evident.

4.18 How is stress echocardiography performed?

BASIC PRINCIPLES

This technique assesses cardiac function during exertional or pharmacological stress, and has some advantages and disadvantages over standard approaches to stress testing. Because of the problems associated with movement, pharmacological stress echocardiography is sometimes the preferred approach where positive inotropes and chronotropes (e.g. dobutamine and arbutamine) are given as a continuous intravenous infusion, sometimes augmented by atropine to increase the heart rate further. The contractile performance of the heart is assessed in multiple views, incorporating the sixteen segments of the heart, at rest and during graded stress. Stress echocardiography is, therefore, a demanding technique that requires a rigorous and skilled approach by highly trained operators.

CLINICAL APPLICATION

Stress echocardiography is directed mainly at assessing the development of, or improvement in, myocardial wall motion abnormalities during stress. Deteriorating regional wall motion during increasing stress suggests the development of myocardial ischaemia and underlying CHD. Alternatively, previously akinetic or hypokinetic areas of myocardium can improve during dobutamine stress and may indicate the presence of 'stunned' myocardium where a recent period of profound ischaemia has led to a temporary reduction in contractile function. A combination of features may also exist, where the contractile function initially improves with low dose dobutamine infusion, only to deteriorate at higher doses. This suggests the presence of 'hibernating' myocardium where a critical, flow-limiting coronary artery stenosis causes contractile dysfunction at rest but the myocardium retains the ability to develop short-lived improvement in contractile function with inotropic stimulation before subsequent ischaemic deterioration occurs at higher workloads. A completely unresponsive akinetic segment indicates an area of infarcted myocardium.

As with other forms of stress testing, stress echocardiography assists in the diagnosis of ischaemic heart disease and guides the use of cardiac catheterisation. It is particularly useful in the management of patients with suspected dynamic or 'hibernating' ischaemic left ventricular dysfunction. Under these circumstances, coronary revascularisation can significantly improve symptoms and left ventricular function.

ASSESSMENT FOR CORONARY ARTERY DISEASE

4.19 Who needs a coronary angiogram?

Cardiac catheterisation is performed in a diagnostic imaging suite as an elective outpatient day case procedure or as an emergency in hospitalised patients with clinical instability. The assessment for coronary artery disease is the main indication (*Box 4.1*) although it is employed in many other conditions including valvular heart disease and heart failure.

BOX 4.1 Indications for coronary angiography

■ Acute myocardial infarction: primary percutaneous coronary intervention, refractory post infarct symptoms, treatment of complications such as acquired ventricular septal defect
■ Unstable angina: refractory symptoms, high risk clinical features
■ Stable angina: refractory symptoms, high risk clinical features
■ Severe asymptomatic ischaemia

The catheterisation procedure is performed through a peripheral artery. The right femoral artery is the most commonly used route because it facilitates imaging in a greater range of views, is more convenient and has a wider calibre. The brachial or radial artery may be used in preference to the femoral artery, particularly when the patient has a coarctation of the aorta, severe peripheral vascular disease or is being treated with anticoagulant therapy.

4.20 When should a coronary angiogram be considered in patients with stable CHD?

In patients with stable coronary artery disease, coronary angiography should be considered where coronary revascularisation may have a role in improving symptoms or prognosis. Coronary angiography is also appropriate in patients in whom non-invasive tests have been inconclusive or negative, but who continue to have chest pain which is severe, frequent or results in recurrent admission to hospital.

The severity of symptoms indicating the need for coronary angiography will vary depending on the patient's (and doctor's) perception of their illness. However, most experts agree that patients with symptoms in Canadian Cardiovascular Society Class 3 or 4 (symptoms on minimal exertion or at rest, *see Box 2.1*) despite adequate medical therapy should be offered angiography as they may benefit from coronary revascularisation.

There are a number of clinical and investigational indicators that identify patients who are at relatively high risk. The threshold for considering coronary angiography should therefore be lower in these patients compared with those being considered purely on the basis of their symptoms because coronary revascularisation may confer prognostic benefits.

4.21 When should a coronary angiogram be considered in patients with unstable CHD?

Coronary angiography with a view to coronary revascularisation should be considered in all patients presenting with an acute coronary syndrome.

In acute ST segment elevation myocardial infarction (*see Ch. 9*), percutaneous coronary intervention is associated with better clinical outcomes and survival when compared to intravenous thrombolytic therapy. The widespread use of this treatment for acute myocardial infarction is limited by the availability and resource implications of this expensive specialised treatment.

During the in-hospital phase of recovery from myocardial infarction or unstable angina, coronary angiography should be considered in high-risk patients, such as those with elevations in cardiac markers, extensive electrocardiographic changes or the development of left ventricular failure.

An initial invasive strategy of coronary angiography with a view to coronary revascularisation is associated with a reduction in readmission with recurrent myocardial ischaemia, myocardial infarction and death.

4.22 What is the role of non-invasive CT scanning in the diagnosis of CHD?

Non-invasive computed tomography is increasingly being employed as a screening method for CHD. This technique generally employs electron beam or multislice systems to image the contracting heart. It is the increased rapidity of the acquisition times that enables these modern scanners to assess the coronary artery tree without movement artefact.

The presence of calcification within the coronary arteries is used as evidence of coronary atherosclerosis (*Fig. 4.6*). Atherosclerosis of the coronary arterial tree is an early and common phenomenon. It is detectable in a third of apparently healthy 30 to 40-year-old individuals and is almost universal once over the age of 70 years. Many people are able to tolerate a large atherosclerotic plaque burden without apparent coronary arterial luminal encroachment through the process of arterial or 'Glagovian' remodelling where the artery expands to accommodate the plaque. Thus,

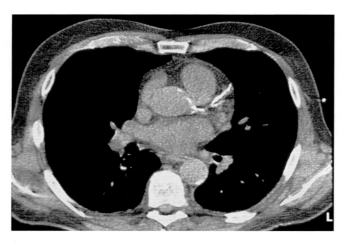

▲

Fig. 4.6 Coronary artery calcification. Ultrafast CT image of coronary calcification. In this transaxial plane the calcium deposited in the coronary arteries can be seen in the wall of the aorta, the left main stem, the left anterior descending coronary artery, and the first diagonal branch.

luminal stenosis causing haemodynamic flow limitation is a late phenomenon and does not occur in the majority of subjects. Therefore, the presence of coronary calcification is associated with coronary atherosclerosis but this does not mean that a patient has, or will develop, clinically evident CHD.

When comparing angiographic evidence of coronary stenoses with the presence of coronary calcification on computed tomography, the sensitivity is excellent but the specificity is poor. Therefore, the absence of calcification is helpful but the presence of vascular calcification does not necessarily confer a diagnosis of CHD.

Risk factors for CHD

5

CHOLESTEROL

5.1 Is cholesterol a risk factor for coronary artery disease?

Raised cholesterol is one of the most important risk factors for coronary heart disease (CHD). A recent study examined selected major risk factors and the global and regional burden of disease.[1] The study reviewed evidence from published work, government reports and international databases to obtain data on the prevalence of risk factor exposure and hazard for 14 epidemiological regions worldwide. In both developing and developed regions, alcohol, tobacco, high blood pressure and high cholesterol were major causes of disease burden. Indeed, the most recent data suggest that cholesterol concentrations exceeding 3.8 mmol/L account for 18% of strokes and 55% of CHD.[2] Treatment of high blood pressure and high cholesterol in individuals with a CHD risk of >35% over 10 years is highly cost effective by averting 63 million disability adjusted life years worldwide.

5.2 What is the evidence for this risk?

Cholesterol is an important cause of CHD, even in patients with average cholesterol levels. Observational studies demonstrate that there is a continuous relationship between risk of CHD and serum cholesterol which is roughly linear. Therefore, a sustained difference of 1 mmol/L in cholesterol concentration is associated with an approximately 50% difference in CHD incidence, irrespective of baseline levels. Indeed, the existence of risk factor thresholds for many common risk factors including cholesterol has recently come under scrutiny.[4] The aim of treatment is not, therefore, to normalise risk factors, but to reduce them as much as possible. It is accepted that risk can be reduced by lowering high cholesterol levels by drug therapy. However, it is still believed by many that changing the average value of cholesterol is not worthwhile, a view which implies a threshold of risk. Such views are reinforced by the use of the term 'hypercholesterolaemia' to indicate a disease state. Moreover, clinical guidelines specifying cholesterol thresholds which – although they have been set at progressively lower levels – still deny some patients effective treatment if their cholesterol is below specified threshold levels.

5.3 Is there a threshold of risk or is it continuous?

Observational studies in different populations indicate a continuous positive relationship between CHD risk and low density lipoprotein (LDL) cholesterol concentration that extends well below the range currently seen in Western populations with no definite 'threshold' below which a lower cholesterol concentration is not associated with a lower CHD risk. Moreover, when the CHD risk is plotted on a logarithmic scale, the relationship is approximately linear, suggesting that the proportional reduction in CHD risk associated with a given absolute reduction in cholesterol is similar over the entire range of cholesterol studied to date. This means that the absolute reduction in CHD risk produced by cholesterol reduction is determined more by the individual's overall risk of CHD rather than just their initial cholesterol concentrations in isolation. This has been clearly demonstrated in the recent MRC/BHF Heart Protection Study in 20 536 high risk individuals.[3] Cholesterol reduction with the HMG CoA reductase inhibitor simvastatin reduced the rates of myocardial infarction by 25% irrespective of the subjects' initial cholesterol concentrations.

5.4 Is treatment beneficial?

Cholesterol reduction has proved to be one of the most effective interventions for the reduction of CHD. A large number of randomised controlled trials have demonstrated a clear reduction in cardiovascular events when cholesterol levels are reduced in patients both with and without coronary disease. Benefits of cholesterol reduction are greatest in patients with known coronary disease as they are at highest risk (*see Q. 5.3*). Recent post-myocardial infarction studies show that subjects with what would previously have been defined as 'normal' or 'average' cholesterol levels also benefit from cholesterol reduction, confirming that there appears to be no threshold of cholesterol below which reduction is not beneficial (*see Q. 5.3*). Moreover, recent data suggest that the use of statins for cholesterol reduction may confer additional benefit beyond that attributable to cholesterol reduction alone. Possible mechanisms include:

- decrease in blood pressure
- anti-inflammatory effects
- improvement in endothelial function
- plaque stabilisation.

Surprisingly, it has recently been shown that cholesterol reduction with statins significantly decreases the incidence of stroke despite no evidence of an epidemiological relationship between cholesterol levels and stroke. This effect of statins may be due to reduction in blood pressure, particularly in the aorta, which has been demonstrated in a number of small trials.

5.5 Who benefits most from treatment?

Since there is no threshold of risk associated with serum cholesterol levels (*see Q. 5.3*), it is clear that individuals at highest risk of a cardiovascular event will benefit most from cholesterol reduction and that the lower the level achieved, the greater the benefit.

Diabetics are at especially high risk of CHD and subgroup analysis of cholesterol reduction trials, which included diabetic subjects, show that diabetics benefit more from cholesterol reduction than non-diabetics, both in primary and secondary prevention trials. Indeed, a recent study shows that type 2 diabetics have the same cardiovascular risk as non-diabetics post-myocardial infarction, suggesting a strong case for all patients with type 2 diabetes to receive cholesterol lowering therapy. Since the benefits of cholesterol reduction are proportional to cardiovascular risk, patients post-myocardial infarction, or with known CHD, will benefit more from cholesterol reduction than patients with raised cholesterol but no clinical evidence of CHD.

A recent global and regional analysis showed that cholesterol reduction in combination with reductions in systolic blood pressure would be highly cost effective and may potentially lower the global incidence of cardiovascular events by as much as 50%.[2]

HYPERTENSION

5.6   Is hypertension a major risk factor for CHD?

The recent global burden of disease study identifies hypertension as the third most common cause of morbidity and mortality.[1] Indeed, hypertension is a powerful independent risk factor for all clinical manifestations of atheromatous disease including CHD, stroke, peripheral vascular disease and heart failure (*Fig. 5.1*).[5] Compared to age- and gender-matched normotensive individuals, the rate of cardiovascular events is approximately two- to four-fold higher in individuals with hypertension. Although the risks attributable to raised blood pressure are greater for heart failure than for coronary disease, the most common sequela of hypertension is CHD, due to its greater incidence in the general population (*see Fig. 1.2*). The disappointing results from large trials of antihypertensive therapy in terms of preventing CHD cast some doubt as to the importance of hypertension and development of CHD. However, the relationship between the severity of hypertension and the development of CHD is strong in all population-based studies.

The fact that atheroma seldom occurs in vessels exposed to low blood pressure (e.g. veins) strengthens the view that raised blood pressure is critical to the atherogenic process. Recently high normal blood pressure (130–139/85–89 mmHg) has been associated with significant risk in both men and women[6] and, since blood pressure in this range is considerably more common than some more severe forms of hypertension, a large proportion of the cardiovascular disease attributable to hypertension derives from this level of blood pressure previously thought to be innocuous.

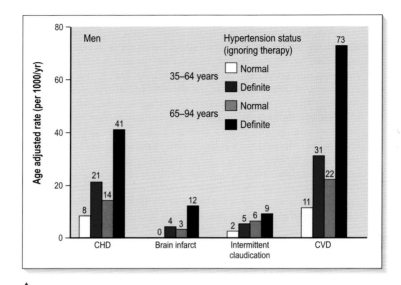

Fig. 5.1 Age-adjusted annual rate of CHD according to hypertension status in the Framingham Heart Study: 30 year follow-up. CVD, cardiovascular disease. (Adapted from Izzo and Black,[5] with permission from Lippincott Williams & Wilkins.)

The high prevalence of hypertension world-wide and its impact on the incidence of CHD, coupled with the large evidence base on the benefits of blood pressure reduction, justify increased efforts to detect and treat raised blood pressure in all populations world-wide. Indeed, systolic blood pressure above 115 mmHg accounts for two-thirds of strokes and about half of CHD world-wide and for cholesterol concentrations of >3.8 mmol/L for 18% and 55%, respectively.[2]

5.7 Which component of blood pressure is most important?

With age, the relative predictive value of the various blood pressure components changes. In younger subjects (<50 years) diastolic pressure best predicts risk, whereas in older subjects systolic and pulse pressure are more important.[7] Indeed, in the elderly systolic hypertension is the predominant form of hypertension, and results from large artery stiffening rather than increased peripheral vascular resistance. In such patients treatment of elevated systolic blood pressure, whether isolated or accompanied by raised diastolic blood pressure, greatly reduces the risk of CHD. Therefore, over-reliance on diastolic blood pressure to assess hypertensive risk is misleading, especially in populations where the predominant form of hypertension is systolic hypertension. Indeed, some experts have advocated the abandonment of diastolic blood pressure altogether.[8] Although a number of studies support pulse pressure as a good predictor of CHD, the relative importance of pulse pressure versus systolic blood pressure as a predictor of CHD remains uncertain. However, increased pulse pressure is a better surrogate marker of large arterial stiffness, itself an independent predictor of CHD. As the large arteries stiffen with age, central blood pressure rises due to increased pressure wave reflection from the periphery and the predictive value of central blood pressure measurements has recently been demonstrated. With the advent of modern technology, the central aortic arterial pressure waveform can now be reconstructed non-invasively from the radial artery waveform[9] (*Fig. 5.2*). In the future therefore, accurate analysis of the central pressure waveform is likely to provide more information in terms of CHD risk stratification than clinic-based measurements of peripheral blood pressure, and central blood pressure may turn out to become the most important component of blood pressure in terms of CHD risk.

5.8 What is the prevalence of CHD in hypertensive subjects?

Coronary heart disease and its sequelae are two to four times more prevalent in patients with hypertension than in normotensive individuals of the same age. The prevalence of CHD in hypertensives increases dramatically if other cardiovascular risk factors such as smoking, hypercholesterolaemia or diabetes are also present. Although hypertension imposes a greater risk for heart failure and less for CHD, because of the greater incidence of CHD in the general population, coronary disease is the most common adverse event associated with hypertension.

5.9 Why is CHD common in hypertensives?

The fact that CHD is common among patients with high blood pressure is well established but the pathophysiological mechanisms underlying this association have until recently been poorly understood. It is now clear that hypertension rarely occurs in isolation and is often associated with one or more risk factors including dyslipidaemia, glucose intolerance, abdominal obesity and hyperinsulinaemia. Recent data from the Framingham study indicate that the prevalence of hypertension in the absence of other risk factors for CHD was <20%. Indeed, 63% of CHD occurring in hypertensive men was associated with two or more additional risk factors (*Table 5.1*). The clustering of two or three major risk factors with hypertension was found to occur at a rate of 50%, twice the rate that could be attributable to chance alone. The CHD risk in both men and women in the Framingham study increased with the number of additional risk factors such that 39% of

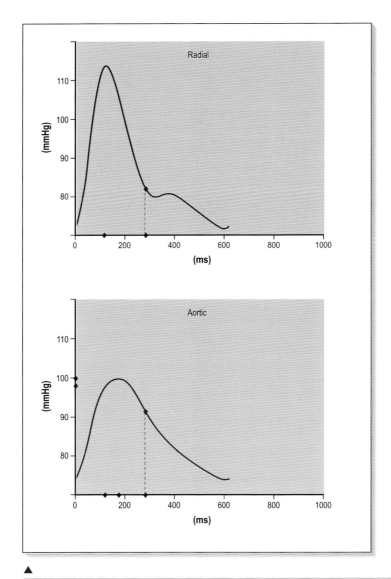

▲

Fig. 5.2 Non-invasive aortic waveform derived using pulse wave analysis. Radial waveforms are recorded using applanation tonometry and then a transfer function is used to derive an ascending aortic waveform. Note the difference in systolic pressure.

TABLE 5.1 Number of other risk factors in hypertensives				
	Percentage with risk factors		Observed/expected ratio	
Number of risk factors	Men	Women	Men	Women
0	24.4	19.5	0.74	0.59
1	29.1	28.1	0.71	0.69
≥2	46.5	52.4	1.8	2.01

Data from Framingham Heart Study offspring. Subjects 18–65 years old. Adapted from Izzo and Black.[5]

coronary events in men with hypertension was attributable to clustering of two or more risk factors.

5.10 Should blood pressure be treated in patients with CHD?

Blood pressure should be treated aggressively in patients with CHD, the major aim of which is to reduce the risk of myocardial infarction and stroke. Hypertensive patients with established CHD are at a considerable risk of myocardial infarction or other major coronary events. In addition, such patients are also at increased risk of death following an acute myocardial infarction. This can be explained, in part, by the fact that hypertension increases myocardial oxygen demand due to the increased output impedance to left ventricular ejection and is a common cause of left ventricular hypertrophy, itself an independent risk factor for CHD. Coupled with the decreased myocardial perfusion and oxygen supply associated with CHD, this substantially increases the risk of CHD. β-blockers not only reduce blood pressure but also improve symptoms of angina and improve mortality; they should therefore be the drug of choice in patients with hypertension and coexisting coronary artery disease and in stable angina.

5.11 What level of blood pressure should be treated?

The levels of blood pressure that should be treated to reduce the risk of CHD come from evidence-based guidelines compiled by expert committees using data from large, well-constructed blood pressure reduction trials. The recommended treatment levels based on the current British Hypertension Society guidelines[10] are summarised in *Figure 5.3*, as are those from the USA[11] (*Table 5.2*).

It is important to recognise the increased risk in patients with diabetes and also the fact that other cardiovascular risk factors tend to cluster in patients with hypertension. Recently, it has become clear that even patients with high normal blood pressure (130–139/85–89 mmHg) are at increased risk of CHD. This finding has led the latest American guidelines (JNC VII)[11] to introduce the term pre-hypertension (120–139/80–89 mmHg). Their recommendations for subjects in this group is to introduce lifestyle modification and reduce their other associated risk factors initially and to introduce drug therapy only if blood pressure becomes raised >140/90 mmHg.

Borderline hypertension
There is a strong association between raised blood pressure and CHD risk even before the development of established hypertension. Borderline (non-sustained) hypertension occurs when the blood pressure is >140/90 mmHg at the initial assessment, but such elevation is neither excessive nor persistent. A major category of patients would be one that exhibits elevated clinic blood pressure readings but not elevated out-of-office readings (white coat hypertension). When blood pressure measurements are repeated, <30% of patients with borderline hypertension remain hypertensive. However, the prognosis for individuals who only have occasional blood pressures >149/90 mmHg is not normal; over a 20-year period their risk of CHD is four-fold greater than normotensive individuals. Such patients also carry an increased risk of developing sustained hypertension in later life. In such patients it is vital to obtain home blood pressure readings either with a validated automatic device (two readings per day for 1 week) or 24 hour ambulatory blood pressure monitoring. There is much epidemiological data on clinic blood pressure measurements and CHD risk but little on home blood pressure measurements and CHD risk. The upper limit of borderline hypertension is 131/83 mmHg for men and 121/78 mmHg for women.

5.12 Do patients with CHD benefit more or less from blood pressure reduction?

Patients with established CHD are likely to benefit more from blood pressure reduction than those without CHD due to the higher initial risks. However, although the majority of studies show a continuous relationship between diastolic blood pressure and CHD risk, some studies suggest that there is a J-shaped curve in that below a diastolic pressure of 85 mmHg the risk of a myocardial infarction increases. The Hypertension Optimal Treatment (HOT) trial did show a small increase in myocardial infarction and cardiovascular mortality at a diastolic pressure <80 mmHg. Since myocardial blood flow occurs mostly in diastole, patients with CHD are less tolerant of a low diastolic pressure and it may therefore be wise to

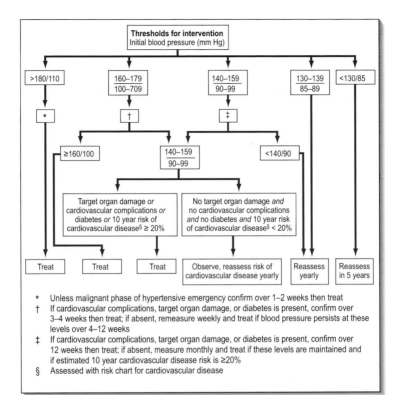

Fig. 5.3 British Hypertension Society guidelines for hypertension management 2004 (BHS-IV). Blood pressure thresholds for intervention. (Adapted from Williams et al.[10] with permission from the BMJ Publishing Group.)

avoid lowering diastolic blood pressure <80 mmHg in patients with significant CHD.

5.13 Does blood pressure reduction reduce the risk of myocardial infarction?

The predicted benefit of lowering blood pressure on the incidence of stroke should be a 35–40% reduction, and evidence from large trials demonstrates an observed reduction of 42 ± 6%, suggesting a direct relationship between stroke and blood pressure. For myocardial infarction, however, the relationship to blood pressure is more complex. A decrease in myocardial

TABLE 5.2 JNC 7 guidelines for the treatment of hypertension in the USA

BP classification	Systolic blood pressure (mmHg)	Diastolic blood pressure (mmHg)	Lifestyle modification	Drug treatment
Normal	<120	and <80	Encourage	No
Prehypertension	120–139	or 80–89	Yes	No
Stage 1 hypertension	140–159	or 90–99	Yes	Yes
Stage 2 hypertension	≥160	or ≥100	Yes	Yes

Adapted from the Seventh Report of the Joint National Committee (JNC 7).[11]

infarction of 20–25% would be predicted but, unlike stroke, the blood pressure trials have demonstrated only a $14 \pm 5\%$ reduction. The lower than expected efficacy of antihypertensive therapy for the prevention of CHD has led to speculation as to the aetiological role of hypertension in the development of CHD. However, in population-based studies, risk of CHD is related to the severity of the antecedent hypertension. Moreover, it would appear that blood pressure is vital to the development of atheroma as this condition rarely occurs in low pressure circulation such as the venous system. In addition, other risk factors for CHD such as diabetes and hypercholesterolaemia often co-segregate with hypertension and, at least in the early trials, subjects with diabetes were often excluded which may account to some extent for the gap between predicted and observed benefits in terms of myocardial infarction.

DIABETES

5.14 Is diabetes a risk factor for CHD?

Diabetes is a major risk factor for the development of CHD. Indeed, diabetes is associated with a two- to four-fold increase in the risk of developing CHD, and patients with diabetes but no clinical evidence of CHD have the same risk of myocardial infarction as non-diabetic patients post myocardial infarction. In patients with diabetes and CHD the death rate is approximately 45% over 7 years and 75% over 10 years.[12]

5.15 Why is CHD more common in diabetes?

The exact pathophysiological mechanisms which increase CHD risk in patients with diabetes remain unclear. Part of the risk may be explained by the clustering of other risk factors such as hypertension and dyslipidaemia with diabetes in the so-called 'metabolic syndrome'. However, this alone is insufficient to explain the high rate of CHD seen in patients with diabetes. As a result, many clinicians and researchers now regard diabetes as a vascular disease. Indeed, the fact that many risk factors for CHD are present long before the development of diabetes has led to increasing support for the 'common soil' hypothesis in which type 2 diabetes and CHD share common genetic and environmental antecedence. Although at a cellular level the various mechanisms linking the metabolic syndrome, type 2 diabetes and atherosclerosis have not as yet been clarified, at a physiological level there is a common pathophysiological abnormality, i.e. endothelial dysfunction characterised by decreased bioavailability of the anti-atherogenic molecule nitric oxide.

5.16 What is syndrome X?

It remains unclear why individuals with type 2 diabetes have such a high incidence of cardiovascular disease. It has been suggested that it may be due to clustering of additional risk factors in such patients. Common additional risk factors are hypertension, insulin resistance, dyslipidaemia and obesity, which together have been termed the 'metabolic syndrome X'. This is distinct from the 'cardiac syndrome X' where there is typical anginal chest pain, a positive stress test but angiographically normal coronary arteries. Interestingly, there is a high prevalence of metabolic syndrome X in patients with cardiac syndrome X.

5.17 Is there a threshold of risk?

Similar to hypertension and hypercholesterolaemia, recent evidence would suggest that there is no threshold of risk. Indeed, in the Norfolk cohort of the European Prospective Investigation into Cancer and Nutrition (EPIC-Norfolk) study, glycosylated haemoglobin concentration was a continuous risk factor throughout the whole population distribution. Such findings emphasise the importance of population-based strategies, not only to treat individuals with established diabetes but also to prevent it where possible by reducing obesity in the general population as a major target.

5.18 Is treatment beneficial?

A number of risk factors such as hypertension and dyslipidaemia are more common in subjects with diabetes, especially type 2 diabetes. The UK Prospective Diabetes Study (UKPDS) addressed the issue of tight blood pressure and tight blood sugar control in the large cohort of newly diagnosed type 2 diabetics. Tight blood pressure control was more effective than tight blood sugar control in terms of reducing both myocardial infarction and stroke. However, individuals with type 2 diabetes are at a greater risk of CHD than non-diabetics and thus will obtain greater absolute risk reduction even if antihypertensive therapy produces the same relative risk reduction as it does in non-diabetic subjects. Indeed, data from the Systolic Hypertension Evaluation Programme (SHEP) study demonstrated that the 583 diabetic patients included in the study obtained twice the absolute risk reduction in CHD compared with non-diabetic subjects. Again due to the higher baseline risk of CHD, diabetics with raised cholesterol concentrations also benefited more from cholesterol reduction than non-diabetics. Indeed, the most recent evidence from the MRC/BHF Heart Protection study which involved 5963 individuals with diabetes provides direct evidence that cholesterol lowering is beneficial for subjects with diabetes even if they do not already have manifest CHD or high cholesterol concentration.[13] In this study, treatment with the HMG CoA reductase inhibitor simvastatin decreased the rate of first major vascular events by approximately 25% across a wide range of diabetic patients studied. The trialists suggested that statin therapy should now be considered routinely for all diabetic patients at significantly high risk of CHD, irrespective of their initial cholesterol concentrations.

Overall, the best approach to reducing CHD risk in subjects with diabetes is probably aggressive, multiple risk factor intervention that targets smoking, hyperglycaemia, hypertension, dyslipidaemia, exercise and diet. This approach has recently been tested in the STENNO 2 trial[14] in which multiple risk factor intervention was compared to usual care. The group receiving multiple risk factor intervention had a 50% reduction in cardiovascular events.

5.19 Who benefits most from treatment?

Individuals with type 2 diabetes are at greater risk of a cardiovascular event than non-diabetics and will thus obtain a greater absolute risk reduction, even if treatment produces a similar relative risk reduction as it does in subjects without diabetes. Diabetic subjects with coexisting hypertension and/or hyperlipidaemia stand to gain most benefit provided blood pressure and cholesterol are aggressively lowered to evidence-based targets. Indeed, the 583 subjects with diabetes in the SHEP study obtained twice the absolute risk reduction in cardiovascular events compared to non-diabetic subjects. Similarly, in the SYSTEUR study there was a greater relative risk reduction in the 492 subjects with diabetes treated with a long-acting calcium channel blocker than in the non-diabetic group. To date, evidence also indicates that elderly diabetics benefit more from treatment. This is supported by the results of the SYSTEUR study where the largest reduction in cardiovascular events was seen in the elderly diabetic population.

Diabetics with coexisting renal disease are also at extremely high cardiovascular risk, and blood pressure reduction in this group of patients has been shown to be extremely beneficial. Interestingly, there is now evidence to suggest that the use of either ACE inhibition or angiotensin II receptor antagonism as blockade of the renin–angiotensin system appears to confer benefit beyond blood pressure reduction alone in this high risk patient cohort. The effect of aggressive cholesterol reduction in this group is as yet unclear but it is currently the subject of a number of ongoing intervention trials.

LIFESTYLE FACTORS

5.20 What are the lifestyle factors that increase the risk of CHD?

Although hypertension, diabetes and hypercholesterolaemia are all major independent risk factors for CHD, accounting for much cardiovascular morbidity and mortality, a number of potentially modifiable lifestyle factors also influence the risk of CHD. These include obesity, lack of exercise, smoking and poor diet. Moreover, intensive lifestyle intervention has been shown to be beneficial. In the Lifestyle Heart Trial,[15] 1 year of comprehensive lifestyle changes (low-fat vegetarian diet, stopping smoking, stress management training and moderate exercise) showed regression of CHD (as assessed by quantitative angiography) in 82% of this group. In contrast, in the control group angiographic lesions were seen to progress. However, as yet there are no data concernign mortality benefit.

5.21 What is the evidence for obesity?

Data from the Framingham Heart Study with a follow-up of more than 20 years show a clear relationship between body weight and the incidence of CHD. Indeed, cardiovascular disease is a major cause of morbidity and mortality among obese individuals. In the prospective Nurses' Health Study[16] involving 115 195 women over 18 years of follow up, death from CHD was higher in the obese (BMI >29 kg/m^2) (*Fig. 5.4*). However, it is still unclear as to whether obesity per se increases the risk of CHD or whether its effect is mediated via other cardiovascular risk factors such as diabetes, hypertension and dyslipidaemia which tend to co-segregate with obesity. Evidence for a direct link between obesity and CHD comes from epidemiological studies. The Framingham study used multivariate analysis to control for other cardiovascular risk factors, and confirmed a relationship between severe and even mild to moderate overweight and CHD risk. In addition, left ventricular hypertrophy, considered as a risk factor for CHD, also correlated with BMI. Finally, obesity strongly increases the risk of both type 2 diabetes and hypertension, both independent risk factors for CHD.

5.22 What are the benefits of weight reduction?

Despite a large body of evidence linking obesity to an increased risk of CHD, to date no prospective trial has addressed the issue of whether intensive weight reduction reduces the incidence of CHD. However, several clinical trials have demonstrated that treatment of obesity reduces other coexistent risk factors for CHD including hypertension and hypercholesterolaemia (*Box 5.1*). In both normotensive and hypertensive individuals, weight loss reduces both systolic and diastolic blood pressure to an extent proportional to total weight loss. In a recent study, weight loss achieved using the fat absorption inhibitor orlistat, reduced the incidence of diabetes by 23% in a group of obese, insulin-resistant individuals with impaired glucose tolerance. Weight reduction also decreases cholesterol concentration.

5.23 How can weight loss be achieved?

Treatment for obesity requires a multifold approach directed at changing and maintaining lifestyle. Dietary advice should address total calorific intake, and aim to reduce the proportion of diet made up of highly refined carbohydrates. The goals of weight loss and an ideal target weight should be established with the patient at the outset of a weight loss programme. Depending on the severity of obesity and the degree of patient motivation, a number of different methods are available. Most involve a multifactor approach involving nutritional education, encouragement to moderate alcohol intake, and programmes to promote increased physical activity. Unfortunately, the results of lifestyle modification can be poor, with most trials demonstrating a return to baseline weight within a few years for many patients.

Drug therapy may be appropriate for carefully selected and motivated patients, although the long term usefulness of this approach has not yet been tested. Two of the most promising anti-obesity drugs at present are sibutramine and orlistat, which appear to be very effective in helping patients to achieve and possibly maintain weight reduction. Since patients receiving these drugs require careful selection and close monitoring they remain largely confined to specialist clinics, and are not suitable for use that is more widespread.

5.24 Is alcohol associated with CHD?

Observational epidemiological studies show that low to moderate levels of alcohol intake are associated with a lower incidence of CHD compared with no alcohol consumption. These beneficial effects may be related to a number of metabolic actions of alcohol including increased high density lipoprotein (HDL) cholesterol, increases in apolipoproteins A_1 and A_2, antioxidant effects, decreases in fibrinogen and decreased platelet aggregation. However, excess alcohol intake is associated with hypertension, cardiomyopathy and haemorrhagic and thrombotic strokes. Moreover, data from the Copenhagen City Heart Study[18] suggest that wine drinking may be

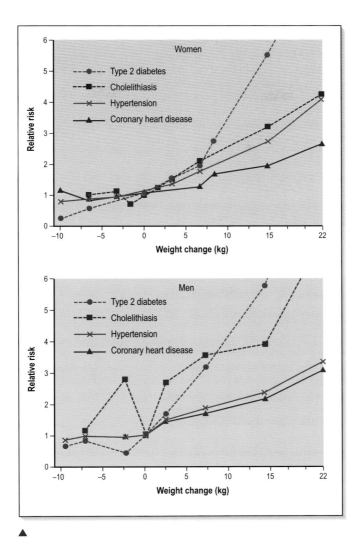

Fig. 5.4 Relation between the change in weight and relative risk of type 2 diabetes, hypertension, coronary heart disease, and cholelithiasis. The upper panel shows these relations for change of weight among women in the Nurses' Health Study, initially 30–55 years of age, who were followed for up to 18 years; the lower panel shows the same relations for change of weight among men in the Health Professionals Follow-up Study, initially 40–65 years of age, who were followed for up to 10 years. (From Willett et al.[17] Copyright © 1999 Massachusetts Medical Society. All rights reserved.)

BOX 5.1 Benefits of weight reduction

Benefits of a 10% weight loss in those weighing 100 kg or more at baseline:

- substantial fall in systolic and diastolic blood pressure
- fall of 10% in total cholesterol
- greater than 50% reduction in the risk of developing diabetes
- a 30–40% fall in diabetes-related deaths
- a 20–25% fall in total mortality

Adapted from Royal College of Physicians of London. Clinical management of obese patients, with particular reference to the use of drugs. London: RCP, 1998.

---

better in terms of reducing CHD risks than drinking beer or spirits, although this may be associated with different patterns of consumption and other lifestyle factors.

5.25 Are non-drinkers at lower risk than drinkers?

The relationship between alcohol consumption and CHD risk is complex (*Fig. 5.5*).[18] A J-shaped curve has been identified in many observational population-based studies and this has been subject to a number of different interpretations. Some have interpreted the data to indicate benefit from moderate alcohol consumption and that this is better than total abstinence. Others have suggested that the abstinent group may include many who are already at high CHD risk and who do not consume alcohol due to specific contraindications or concurrent illness.

5.26 Is diet associated with CHD?

The first evidence that diet may be associated with CHD came from studies in the 1970s. The Seven Countries study showed a direct correlation between dietary fat, total cholesterol levels and coronary-related death. Other studies have shown reduced CHD in populations where the diet is low in fat but high in fibre. However, such findings are not universal and data from the Harvard School of Public Health collected over a period of 20 years failed to show any relationship between fat intake and CHD risk. Indeed, some fats such as olive oil and other monounsaturated fats can reduce CHD risk. A number of other epidemiological studies have demonstrated reduced CHD risk from diets high in fatty fish or antioxidant vitamins. However, although epidemiological studies are important, they are not able to establish a causal link between diet and CHD risk.

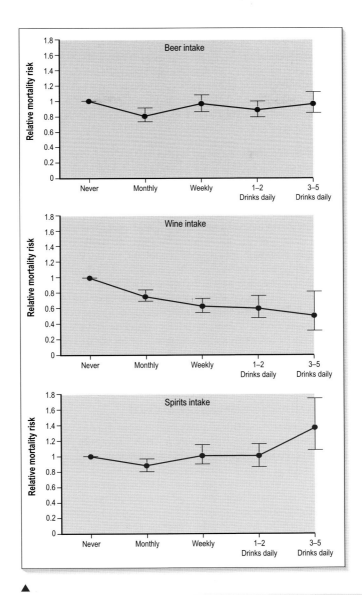

Fig. 5.5 Relative mortality risk associated with frequency of alcohol consumption, for beer, wine, and spirits intake. Data from the Copenhagen City Heart Study. (From Gronbaek et al.[18] with permission from the BMJ Publishing Group.)

5.27 Does dietary intervention decrease the risk of CHD?

Because of the belief that outcome studies are not feasible for dietary interventions, the field has been dominated by small intervention studies measuring intermediate and surrogate endpoints. Although such studies have provided evidence of the effects of dietary intervention (*Box 5.2*) on blood pressure, cholesterol and risk of diabetes, there is little direct evidence on which diets will prevent CHD.

5.28 Is lack of exercise associated with CHD?

Physical inactivity is known to be associated with increased CHD risk. Indeed, the American Heart Association has recently added lack of exercise to the list of major risk factors for CHD. The Harvard Alumni study examined the effect of physical activity and all-cause mortality and longevity in 16 936 male Harvard Alumni aged 35–74. Exercise was inversely related to total mortality, predominantly due to CHD or respiratory causes. Interestingly, a study in 1564 women recruited from the Pennsylvania Alumnae study with a mean age of 45.5 years failed to demonstrate any relationship between physical activity and CHD.[19]

The recent study examining major risk factors of global and regional burden of disease confirmed physical inactivity as a major cause of morbidity and mortality, both in developed and developing countries worldwide.[1] The exact mechanisms responsible for the increased risk of CHD associated with physical inactivity were unclear, but may well involve increased levels of obesity, hypertension and hypercholesterolaemia in subjects who take little exercise.

5.29 Does exercise decrease the risk of CHD?

Many studies have now shown that physical activity, particularly during leisure, is associated with a reduction in CHD.[20] However, the optimal intensity of exercise is unclear. This is especially important as early data from the Harvard Alumni study suggested a J-shaped curve. This was recently addressed in a cohort of 1975 men aged between 49 and 64 years from the Caerphilly Heart study. Light and moderate intensity exercise had inconsistent and non-significant relations to CHD in contrast to significant dose response as seen for heavy intensity exercise and decreased CHD mortality.[21] This finding has also been confirmed by data from the Harvard Alumni study.[22] In addition, this study also showed that there was no difference between longer sessions of exercise compared to shorter ones provided that the total energy expenditure was similar. Doctors should therefore encourage patients to be physically active to decrease their risk of CHD.

Data suggest that physical activity does not have to be arduously long to be beneficial, even short (15 min) sessions appear to confer benefits. The

BOX 5.2   Dietary intervention

Low-fat diets

The Cochrane Collaboration recently published a meta-analysis of 27 randomised intervention trials (40 intervention arms), lasting for at least 6 months. No significant effect was shown with reduced or modified dietary fat on cardiovascular mortality or cardiovascular events (Hooper et al. Cochrane database systemic review 2001;3:CD002137). The Diet and Re-infarction Trial (DART) randomised 2033 men post-myocardial infarction to receive or not receive the following recommendations:

1. Decreased fat intake to 30% of total energy with increased polyunsaturated fat ratio
2. At least two portions of fatty fish weekly
3. Increased fibre intake to 18 g daily.

Two years' advice on dietary fat and fibre intake had no effect on cardiac events.

In terms of primary prevention, the Multiple Risk Factor Intervention Trial (MRFIT) randomised 12 866 men with risk of CHD to receive an intervention that included advice about diet (saturated fat <8% of total energy intake). There was no evidence that a lower fat intake had any effect on CHD.

Antioxidants

Antioxidants have also been proposed for both primary and secondary prevention of CHD. Several large prospective cohort randomised control studies have, however, shown no benefit from β-carotene, vitamin E, vitamin C, selenium or multivitamin supplements in reducing the risk of CHD.

Omega-3 fatty acids

Perhaps the most promising dietary intervention is omega-3 fatty acid supplementation. In the GISSI-Prevenzione trial, patients post myocardial infarction who took fish oil had a decreased incidence of death and non-fatal myocardial infarction relative to controls.

DASH diet

The Dietary Approaches to Stop Hypertension (DASH) trial (*NEJM* 2001;344:3–10) randomised 459 subjects to one of three diets:

1. A typical US diet
2. A diet rich in fruits and vegetables but otherwise similar to control
3. A diet rich in fruit and vegetables and low fat dairy products and low in saturated and total fat (the DASH diet).

BOX 5.2 Dietary intervention—cont'd

Subjects consuming the DASH diet, whether hypertensive or not, showed a significant reduction in blood pressure. Therefore, it would be surprising if the DASH diet had no effect on CHD events. However, the only way that this could be tested would be to routinely assign a group of subjects to the DASH diet versus control and to measure outcome in the two groups.

---

benefits of exercise on CHD risk may also be mediated by the indirect effects of exercise in reducing other CHD risk factors such as hypertension and hypercholesterolaemia. In addition, exercise improves insulin sensitivity and delays or prevents the onset of type 2 diabetes.

Finally, increased arterial stiffness has emerged as a major independent risk factor for CHD and exercise has been shown to decrease arterial stiffness both acutely and chronically.

5.30 What type of exercise is best?

Activity that reduces the risk of CHD does not require a structured or vigorous exercise programme. Major benefits accrue from performing moderate-intensity exercise. At least 120 minutes per week of moderate intensity exercise such as brisk walking appears to be necessary for clinically relevant benefit. Since the frequency, intensity and duration of exercise are interrelated, low intensity or shorter duration exercise should be performed more often to achieve cardiovascular benefit.

5.31 What are the risks of exercise for patients with CHD?

Because the risks of physical activity are very low compared to the resultant health benefits, the majority of individuals do not require medical consultation before embarking on a moderate-intensity exercise programme. However, those with known CHD and men over 40 years and women over 50 years with multiple cardiovascular risk factors require medical evaluation before starting on a programme of exercise. The aim of the medical consultation, which should include a full history and examination, is to determine whether there are any specific medical conditions that are contraindications to exercise such as acute ischaemia, arrhythmias and acute infections. Relative contraindications include valvular heart disease, advanced congestive heart failure, ventricular aneurysm and electrolyte imbalance. However, the risk of serious cardiac events associated with exercise as part of a cardiac rehabilitation programme is reported as very low.[23]

5.32 Is smoking associated with CHD?

Smoking is a major risk factor for CHD and is in the top three causes of death and morbidity world-wide.[1] There is clear dose–response in terms of smoking and CHD risk, and recently the apolipoprotein E4 genotype has been shown to further increase the risk of CHD in male smokers. Passive smoking is also associated with an increased risk of CHD. A recent meta-analysis of epidemiological studies between 1966 and 1988 demonstrated that non-smokers exposed to passive smoking had an overall increased risk of CHD of 25% compared with non-smokers not exposed to passive smoking.[24] Moreover, the risk of CHD increased with exposure to a higher level or longer duration of passive smoking. Although the importance of smoking as a risk factor for CHD is beyond doubt, the speed and magnitude of risk reduction when a smoker with CHD gives up smoking are not clear. Those who quit smoking can expect a reduction of about 36% in mortality compared to those who continue to smoke. Moreover, the risk reduction associated with stopping smoking was consistent regardless of age, sex, country and time period.

5.33 Is anything effective in helping patients to stop smoking?

Both nicotine replacement and amfebutamone (Zyban) are moderately effective in increasing the success rate of smoking cessation programmes. Both are available in the UK for suitable patients.

RENAL FAILURE

5.34 Are patients with end-stage renal failure at risk of CHD?

Patients with end stage renal failure on dialysis have a disproportionately high incidence of CHD. In addition, patients with end stage renal failure suffer increased mortality post myocardial infarction compared to the general population. They also have a significantly higher incidence of acute coronary syndromes. Despite this, recent data show a dramatic underprescription of cardioprotective drugs, such as statins, in this patient population.

Recently, arterial stiffness has emerged as a powerful predictor of cardiovascular risk. Assessment of large artery stiffness by means of measuring aortic pulse wave velocity (PWV) has been shown to be a strong independent predictor of cardiovascular mortality in patients with end-stage renal failure[25,26] (Fig. 5.6). Measurement of aortic PWV in patients with end-stage renal failure, therefore, provides improved prognostic information over and above assessment of conventional cardiovascular risk factors.

5.35 Is treatment beneficial?

The majority of subjects with end-stage renal failure have hypertension. In patients without renal failure blood pressure reduction is effective in reducing cardiovascular events irrespective of the antihypertensive agent used, and the same would appear to be true in patients with renal failure. However, recent data suggest that antihypertensive drugs that reduce arterial stiffness as well as blood pressure may confer additional survival benefits.

Cholesterol reduction has been clearly demonstrated to reduce cardiovascular events in subjects without end-stage renal failure who have pre-existing CHD. Cholesterol reduction also reduces the incidence of CHD in high risk patients. Despite this, statins appear to be underused in patients with end-stage renal failure. However, a number of large studies are currently underway to evaluate the benefits of cholesterol reduction with statins in patients with end-stage renal failure.

5.36 Is the choice of drug important?

Large artery stiffness as assessed by aortic PWV is an important independent predictor of both overall and cardiovascular mortality in

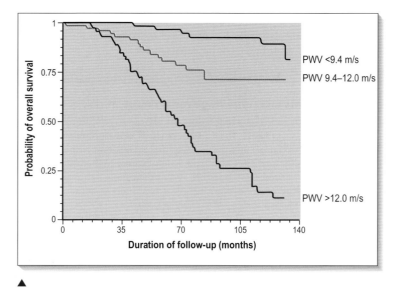

Fig. 5.6 Aortic pulse wave velocity independently predicts mortality in patients with end-stage renal disease. (From Blacher et al.[25] with permission.)

patients with end-stage renal failure. Reduction in mean arterial pressure per se will decrease aortic PWV, but drugs that reduce PWV irrespective of their antihypertensive effect may be expected to be of greater benefit in patients with end-stage renal failure.[27] In addition to aortic PWV, central aortic pressure has also been shown to predict survival in patients with end-stage renal failure. Therefore, drugs that decrease central aortic pressure, such as ACE inhibitors and calcium channel antagonists, may also be beneficial.[3] In addition, ACE inhibitors may also slow the progression of renal decline over and above that due to blood pressure reduction. In contrast, conventional β-blockers such as atenolol have been shown to increase wave reflection from the periphery leading to an increase in central aortic pulse pressure. Such an effect may not be beneficial in patients with end-stage renal failure. With regard to cholesterol reduction, there seems little evidence to suggest differential effects between statins.

5.37 Who benefits most from treatment?

Individuals with the highest aortic PWV and central pulse pressure will be at greatest risk and as such are likely to benefit most from blood pressure reduction. Subjects with pre-existing CHD or diabetes will also be at high risk and, therefore, be likely to obtain greater absolute risk reduction from reduction in blood pressure and cholesterol. The benefits of cholesterol reduction in end-stage renal failure are currently being assessed in large intervention studies.

PRIMARY PREVENTION

5.38 Who should be considered for primary prevention?

The latest Joint British Guidelines recommend that in the primary prevention of CHD, all major risk factors must be considered as they have a cumulative effect on absolute CHD risk (*Box 5.3*).

The absolute risk of developing CHD over the next 10 years is key to determining lifestyle and therapeutic intervention. The intensity of intervention should increase in proportion to absolute risk. It is also important to note that patients will need regular review as CHD risk increases with age. Individuals at highest risk of CHD should be targeted first and it is therefore necessary to identify and treat individuals with >30% risk of CHD over 10 years. However, individuals with CHD risk between 15 and 30% over 10 years will also benefit substantially from blood pressure and cholesterol lowering therapy.

BOX 5.3 Major risk factors to be considered when calculating cardiovascular risk

■ Smoking
■ Blood pressure
■ Total:HDL cholesterol ratio
■ Diabetes
■ Hypertension-related end organ damage, e.g. left ventricular hypertrophy
■ Gender
■ Family history of premature cardiovascular disease

5.39 What treatments should they receive?

■ *Blood pressure*: Individuals at high risk of CHD should have their blood pressure reduced to <140 mmHg systolic and <85 mmHg diastolic pressure. Drug combinations may be required in at least 50% of all hypertensive patients. Drug treatment and combination should be determined by factors such as the age and ethnicity of the individual patient. In those with diabetes, renal disease or cardiovascular disease the target is <130 mmHg and <80 mmHg, and in those with renal disease and proteinuria <125/75 mmHg.

■ *Cholesterol reduction*: A 10% decrease in cholesterol produces an approximately 25% decrease in CHD risk after 2 years' treatment. Results of the primary prevention trials of cholesterol reduction, as with the secondary prevention trial, show no threshold of cholesterol below which further reduction is no longer beneficial. Recommended targets for cholesterol in patients at risk of CHD are <5 mmol/L total cholesterol and <3 mmol/L LDL cholesterol.

■ *Aspirin*: Prophylactic aspirin should be considered in certain high risk individuals. Data for the HOT study show that 75 mg aspirin daily reduces cardiovascular risk in patients with hypertension. The Thrombosis Prevention Trial showed benefits from aspirin in terms of CHD prevention in high risk individuals regardless of blood pressure. Aspirin (75 mg) should therefore be given to individuals over 50 years of age with estimated CHD risk >15% over 10 years unless there is an absolute contraindication. Many clinicians would also give aspirin to subjects with type 2 diabetes and no clinical evidence of CHD as the CHD risk of a type 2 diabetic equates to a non-diabetic post-myocardial infarction.

■ *Diabetes and CHD*: The absolute risk of CHD is greatly increased in patients with diabetes. In type 1 diabetes, the presence of hypertension often reflects the presence of diabetic nephropathy.

> Blood pressure reduction has been shown to slow the rate of declining renal function. ACE inhibitors appear to have a beneficial effect beyond blood pressure reduction alone and should be used as first line therapy in patients with type 1 diabetes, although additional antihypertensive therapy will often be required. Blood pressure targets for diabetics are lower: <130 mmHg systolic and <80 mmHg diastolic pressure. In terms of cholesterol reduction, diabetic patients should receive a statin if their 10 year CHD risk is greater that 15%.

5.40 What are the risks and benefits?

Physiological variables including blood pressure, serum cholesterol and BMI are important factors in the genesis of CHD. Although the mechanisms involved remain poorly understood, it is known that lowering these variables by drug treatment or lifestyle intervention can significantly reduce both cardiovascular risk and events. However, some clinicians and researchers hold the view that decreasing these physiological variables is not worthwhile. This view is reliant on the presence of thresholds in the dose–response relationship between the level of blood pressure or cholesterol for example, and the risk of CHD. Therefore, individuals with raised blood pressure become classified as having a disease 'hypertension'.[4] Despite this, clinical guidelines continue to specify risk factor thresholds although the evidence suggests that no such thresholds exist, especially for hypertension and hypercholesterolaemia. A given change in cholesterol or blood pressure reduces the risk of CHD by a constant proportion of the existing risk irrespective of the starting level of the risk factor or of the existing risk. Interventions to lower blood pressure or cholesterol should therefore be determined by an individual's level of risk, not the level of the risk factors themselves. Indeed, all reversible cardiovascular risk factors should be reduced in anyone at high risk of CHD.

PQ PATIENT QUESTIONS

5.41 Who is at risk of heart disease?

The risk of heart disease increases with age for both men and women. Men are at greater risk than women until women reach the menopause when their risk catches up with that of men. Individuals with a strong family history of premature heart disease (<55 years of age) have an increased risk compared to individuals with no such family history (*see also Q. 5.43*). Much research is now focussing on the genes that may influence heart disease, but as yet this remains unclear.

An unhealthy lifestyle including smoking, high alcohol intake, high fat diet and low levels of physical activity also increases the risk of heart disease. Obesity in the general population is on the rise and this also increases the risk of heart disease, either alone or by increasing the chances of developing diabetes. Individuals with diabetes have a very high incidence of heart disease.

Finally, both high blood pressure and raised blood cholesterol levels significantly increase the risk of heart disease.

5.42 How can I reduce my risk of heart disease?

Lifestyle measures can significantly reduce the risk of coronary heart disease. These include eating at least five portions of fruit or vegetables per day, reducing the amount of saturated fats in the diet, and increasing the dietary intake of oily fish. In addition, decreasing the amount of salt in the diet (under 7 g for men and 5 g for women) helps to keep blood pressure low. Regular exercise and a moderate alcohol intake are also protective against coronary heart disease. In individuals who are obese, losing weight is also likely to be beneficial.

Stopping smoking significantly reduces the risk of coronary heart disease and in individuals who smoke there is a significant reduction in the risk of coronary heart disease within a few years of stopping. It also reduces the risk of lung disease and cancers.

Individuals who have already had a heart attack or who have angina should have their blood pressure and cholesterol checked and treated if necessary.

Finally, individuals over 55 years of age should have their blood pressure and cholesterol checked and if they are overweight with a strong family history of diabetes, they should be screened to make sure that they don't have early diabetes.

5.43 Does heart disease run in families?

There is no doubt that some families have a higher risk of premature heart disease (<55 years of age) than others, even without additional risk factors such as high blood pressure and smoking. The genes that may be responsible for the increased risk of coronary heart disease in some families are being actively looked for at present. However, to date no one gene has been identified and it is likely that many genes will ultimately be involved. If there is a strong family history of coronary heart disease, an individual should make efforts to minimise other additional risk factors such as smoking, inactivity, poor diet, obesity and other lifestyle factors. Just because your parent suffered coronary heart disease at a young age does not necessarily mean that it will definitely happen to you.

5.44   What is a normal cholesterol value?

In patients with angina, or those who have had a heart attack, the cholesterol levels should be below 5.0 mmol/L. However, recent evidence suggests that the lower the cholesterol level the better, and therefore people with 'normal' cholesterol levels will still benefit from cholesterol lowering drugs. Since there appears to be no threshold of risk, the majority of patients with coronary heart disease or at high risk of it, should receive cholesterol lowering medication.

5.45   What is normal blood pressure?

There is a bell-shaped distribution of blood pressure in the general population (just like height varies considerably). The level of blood pressure considered normal is based on epidemiological evidence and evidence from blood pressure reduction trials. Currently, the British Hypertension Society would recommend that individuals with persistently raised blood pressure (>160/100 mmHg) should receive antihypertensive therapy, with target values after treatment of <140/90 mmHg. The threshold for treatment in patients with diabetes is lower with a target value of <130/85 mmHg.

Although systolic blood pressure increases with age in all individuals, a high systolic blood pressure in old age is not, as previously thought, benign and older individuals get more benefit from treatment than younger ones.

Drug treatment for angina

6

Stable angina is caused by an imbalance between oxygen supply to and demand from the myocardium. The aim of treatment for angina is to restore the balance either by increasing myocardial blood flow or by decreasing myocardial oxygen demand (*Fig. 6.1, Box 6.1*). Drug therapy falls into three main categories:

1. Secondary prophylactic treatment
2. Short term control of anginal symptoms
3. Long term prevention of anginal symptoms.

DRUG TREATMENT FOR ANGINA

6.1 Which drug should be used for prophylactic treatment?

ASPIRIN

Aspirin is a cyclo-oxygenase inhibitor which inhibits platelet aggregation (*see Fig. 10.1*). The Swedish Angina Pectoris Aspirin Trial (SAPAT)[1] involved treating 2035 patients with exertional angina with 75 mg aspirin/day. The reduction in the primary endpoint (non-fatal myocardial infarction, fatal myocardial infarction or sudden death) was 35% following 72 months of treatment. Data from the US Physicians Health study also demonstrated that aspirin reduced the risk of a first myocardial infarction in subjects with stable angina. The Antiplatelet Trialists meta-analysis demonstrated clear benefits for patients with coronary heart disease (CHD) treated with aspirin; this group included many individuals with stable angina[2] (*Fig. 6.2*).

In terms of dose, trials have used between 75 and 300 mg daily. However, a recent meta-analysis showed no difference in risk reduction across doses of aspirin from 75 to 500 mg daily. Patients with angina should, therefore, be treated with 75 mg aspirin/day. If patients are genuinely intolerant of aspirin, 75 mg daily of clopidogrel should be considered as an alternative therapy.

STATINS

Statins also have a role in patients with angina, and should be considered in all patients (*see Q. 6.39*).

ACE INHIBITORS

Data from the Heart Outcomes Prevention Evaluation (HOPE) study suggested additional benefits of ACE inhibition beyond blood pressure reduction in patients at high risk of cardiovascular events over the age of 55 years with a history of CHD (*Fig. 6.3*).[3] Recently the EUROPA study also showed benefit from ACE inhibition in a group of low risk patients with stable angina.[4]

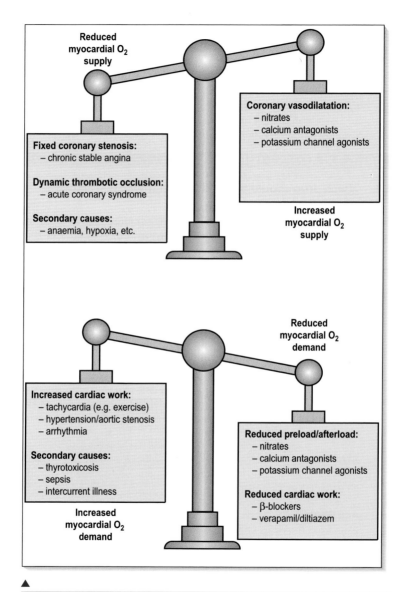

▲

Fig. 6.1 Effect of the main drug classes.

BOX 6.1 Determinants of myocardial oxygen supply and demand

Determinants of myocardial oxygen demand
- Heart rate
- Ventricular contractility
- Myocardial wall tension
- Preload
- Afterload
- Wall thickness
- Metabolic factors

Determinants of myocardial oxygen supply
- Blood flow
- Pressure
- Resistance
- Blood oxygen content and delivery

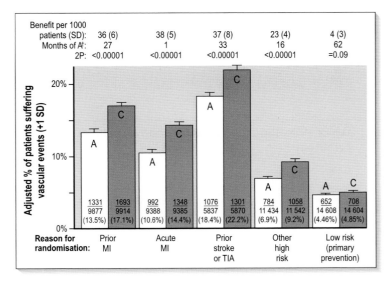

Fig. 6.2 Benefits of aspirin. Absolute effect of aspirin on cardiovascular events in a range of patient groups. Data from 145 trials. A, antiplatelet therapy; C, control; Months of A[†], means of scheduled antiplatelet durations, no trial lasted under 1 month; TIA, transient ischaemic attack. (From Antiplatelet Trialists' Collaboration,[2] with permission from the BMJ Publishing Group.)

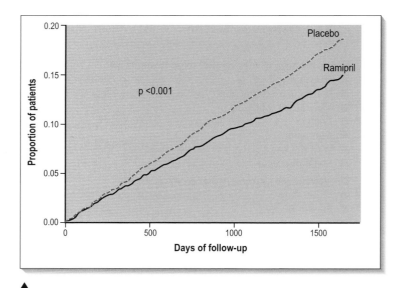

▲

Fig. 6.3 Benefits of ACE inhibitors in patients with coronary heart disease. Kaplan–Meier estimates of the composite outcome of myocardial infarction, stroke or death from cardiovascular causes in the ramipril group and the placebo group. (From Yusuf et al.[3] Copyright © 2000 Massachusetts Medical Society. All rights reserved.)

6.2 Which drug should be used for control and prevention of symptoms?

GTN

Sublingual glyceryl trinitrate (GTN) is the first-line treatment for short term symptom control. It should be remembered that patients should be educated as to its appropriate use, including its prophylactic use in situations where anginal symptoms can be anticipated. They should also be warned of its likely side-effects such as headache and tachycardia and to seek medical advice if pain persists after three doses over 15 minutes.

β-BLOCKERS

β-blockers are as effective in the prevention of long term symptoms as other available drug classes. Data from post myocardial infarction trials and in patients with angina show that β-blockade in high risk patients reduces cardiovascular morbidity and mortality.

Patients who require symptomatic treatment should, therefore, be treated with a β-blocker first line unless contraindicated (*see Q. 6.10*). As there is evidence that in certain patient groups (e.g. those with hypertension) acute withdrawal of β-blockers can increase cardiovascular events, patients should be advised not to stop β-blockers acutely (*see Q. 6.11*). β-blockers are especially useful in patients with coexisting high blood pressure.

CALCIUM CHANNEL BLOCKERS

In patients intolerant of β-blockers or in whom they are contraindicated, calcium channel blockers can be used as an alternative as they have been shown in placebo-controlled trials to be effective first-line agents. However, as yet there is no definitive evidence that any single class of anti-anginal agent is more effective than another. Therefore, patients with contraindications to β-blockade should be treated with a rate limiting calcium channel blocker (*see Q. 6.16*), a long acting dihydropyridine or a nitrate (*see Q. 6.3*).

6.3 Which drug should be used for long term prevention of anginal symptoms?

NITRATES

Oral nitrates are effective anti-anginal agents for long term symptomatic therapy when used as a sustained release preparation. Both isosorbide di- and mononitrate have been shown to be effective in placebo-controlled trials. Nitrate tolerance is a problem (*see Q. 6.20*) and any dose regimen should allow for a 6–8 hour nitrate-free period. There is not a large body of evidence as to the effectiveness of nitrate patches and they are considerably more expensive.

POTASSIUM CHANNEL ACTIVATORS

Potassium channel activators (e.g. nicorandil) are also effective in reducing the symptoms of angina, but seem to offer no particular advantage over other therapies.

Figure 6.4 provides a schema for the drug management of chronic stable angina.

6.4 What is the appropriate interval between assessing response to therapy?

Two weeks would be an appropriate interval before assessing response to therapy both in terms of short and long term prevention of symptoms. If short lived episodes of chest pain are not relieved by sublingual GTN, then alternative diagnoses such as reflux oesophagitis should be considered.

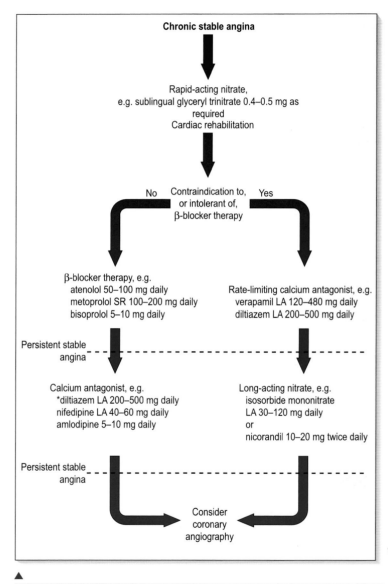

▲

Fig. 6.4 Schema for the symptomatic treatment of patients with chronic stable angina.
*Caution when used in combination with β-blockers as may cause excessive bradycardia.

6.5   Should treatment be cumulative or rotational?

Treatment should probably be cumulative (*see Fig. 6.4*) as no one major class of anti-anginal agent has been shown in a definitive study to be superior to another. However, studies on triple drug combination show no advantage over dual therapy. Indeed, if a patient is not controlled on dual therapy, they should be referred to a cardiologist for further investigation and management (*see Q. 6.7*).

6.6   Which drug combinations are effective?

Evidence from randomised controlled trials supports the use of long acting nitrates or a calcium channel blocker in combination with a β-blocker. However, the combination of diltiazem or verapamil with a β-blocker should be avoided (*see Q. 6.17*). Overall, there is no convincing evidence to support other drug combinations. In practice, however, the use of more than one drug from the same therapeutic class is best avoided. Triple drug combinations do not have any proven advantage over dual therapy and patients who are not controlled on two agents should be referred for further assessment (*see Q. 6.7*).

6.7   Who should be referred for further investigation?

Patients may need referral to a cardiologist either to confirm the diagnosis of CHD or for advice and further management in patients known to have angina and CHD (*Box 6.2*). Such patients may benefit from early investigation or revascularisation.

In addition, patients with a suspected diagnosis of unstable angina – i.e. those presenting with symptoms of pain at rest (which can also occur at night), pain on minimal exertion, and anginal symptoms which are progressing rapidly despite maximal medical therapy – should be referred as a matter of urgency.

β-BLOCKERS

6.8   How do β-blockers work in angina?

The main uses of β-blockers in patients with CHD are in the prophylaxis of angina and in reducing the risk of sudden death or re-infarction following myocardial infarction. β-adrenoceptors are linked via a G-protein to adenyl cyclase, so β-adrenoceptor stimulation leads to an increase in cytoplasmic cyclic adenosine monophosphate (cAMP). In cardiac tissue, cAMP increases force of contraction and heart rate and is arrhythmogenic. β-blockers work by competing with endogenous β-agonists such as adrenaline (epinephrine)

BOX 6.2 Cardiological referral

A cardiological referral is appropriate for patients with stable symptoms who have not previously been assessed and could potentially benefit from further invasive investigation and who have:

- an ECG showing previous myocardial infarction or other significant abnormality suggesting significant ischaemia
- failed to respond to medical therapy and modification of risk factors
- an ejection systolic murmur suggestive of aortic stenosis
- a strong family history and presence of other adverse risk factors
- coexisting diabetes mellitus
- problems with life insurance or employment.

Cardiological referral is also required to confirm the diagnosis in patients with atypical symptoms.

---

and noradrenaline (norepinephrine) and thereby reduce their β-receptor mediated effects (*Box 6.3*). Consequently β-blockers slow the heart and are negatively inotropic. Both these effects lead to a reduction in myocardial oxygen consumption and hence decrease demand. β-blockers have little or no effect on cardiac preload or afterload, although they do increase ejection time which is counterproductive. Although β-blockers have little effect on oxygen supply, the decreased heart rate leads to an increased perfusion time thus increasing oxygen supply to some extent. However, non-selective β-blockers tend to increase coronary artery vasoconstriction due to an α_2-mediated effect which may in some cases offset some of the benefit due to decreased oxygen consumption.

A number of β-blockers have been developed with a degree of selectivity for the β_1 receptors (the predominant type present in cardiac tissue). In addition, a number of β-blockers with partial agonist activity such as oxprenolol and pindolol are also clinically available. Such agents cause a smaller fall in resting heart rate due to their mixed agonist activity, but do prevent further increases in heart rate caused by sympathetic activation such as that occurring during exercise. These agents do not, however, appear to confer any advantage in the clinical treatment of angina and lose the secondary preventative benefits following myocardial infarction.

6.9 What are the indications for their use?

The major indications for the use of β-blockers in angina are the prevention of symptoms and reduction in the risk of sudden death or re-infarction following myocardial infarction. β-blockade is also the treatment of choice in patients with hypertension and coexisting angina due to CHD.

> **BOX 6.3 Beneficial haemodynamic effects of β-blockers in angina**
>
> **Decreased oxygen consumption by:**
> 1. decreased heart rate
> 2. decreased contractility
> 3. no change in preload
> 4. no change in afterload
> 5. increased ejection time (counterproductive).
>
> **Oxygen supply little changed by:**
> 1. decreased heart rate increasing perfusion time (beneficial)
> 2. no change in preload
> 3. a tendency to increase coronary artery constriction (β_2 effect).

β-blockers have been shown to limit infarct size in acute myocardial infarction, and to reduce sudden death. A meta-analysis of 27 randomised trials involving 27 000 patients showed that early intravenous administration followed by oral treatment with a β-blocker reduces mortality by 13% in the first week post-myocardial infarction.[5] When used in conjunction with thrombolytic therapy, β-blockers provide additional benefit, especially if administered early after the onset of symptoms of myocardial infarction.

Benefits of β-blockade appear to persist as long as the drug is continued. It would, therefore, be appropriate to continue β-blockade post-myocardial infarction indefinitely in individuals who can tolerate it. The use of β-blockers in unstable angina has been assessed in a number of small uncontrolled trials, a meta-analysis of which shows a 15% reduction in progression from unstable angina to myocardial infarction, but no significant benefit in terms of reduced mortality.[5]

6.10 What are the contraindications to their use?

In certain patients β-blockade can precipitate bradycardia or atrioventricular blocks. Consequently, they should be given with caution to patients with significant conduction system disease of the sinus or atrioventricular nodes. β-blockers with intrinsic sympathomimetic activity do not appear to decrease resting heart rate as much as β-blockers with no such effect. β-blockers are used extensively in the treatment of hypertension and are known to lower blood pressure. They should, therefore, again be used with caution in patients with low blood pressure. In patients with decreased systolic cardiac function, β-blockers can precipitate heart failure and should be used cautiously. However, once established, β-blockers markedly reduce mortality in patients with heart failure. β-blockers can also precipitate bronchospasm in patients with underlying chronic pulmonary disease via blockade of β_2 receptors. This effect can be diminished by using β_1 selective agents although this effect is relative and tends to decrease at high doses. β-blockers are absolutely contraindicated in patients with asthma.

β-blockers may also lead to a worsening of Raynaud's phenomenon. Again, this effect may be less in agents with a high degree of β_1 selectivity. Finally, it has been suggested that β-blockers may worsen claudication in patients with peripheral vascular disease although this has not been substantiated in controlled trials. If a patient does experience a worsening of claudication, substitution of the β-blocker with intrinsic sympathomimetic activity or a vasodilating β-blocker may be of value. Patients with coronary artery spasm may paradoxically deteriorate on β-blockade due to unopposed α-adrenoceptor mediated vasoconstriction, although this is uncommon.

6.11 What are their adverse effects?

A major cause of adverse effects of β-blockers is their effect on the central nervous system. Such effects include symptoms of fatigue, nightmares and depression. It has been suggested that CNS effects are more common with the more lipophilic β-blockers although there is little evidence to support this.

β-blockers decrease sympathetic activity, and as such may be associated with impotence. A number of metabolic side-effects have also been ascribed to β-blockers. Patients with diabetes may experience mild worsening of glycaemic control and blocking of the symptoms of hypoglycaemia (which are sympathetically mediated), increasing the risk of severe hypoglycaemic attacks. However, the β-blocker atenolol was used in the UKPDS study and there was no evidence that it increased the incidence of severe hypoglycaemia. β-blockers have also been shown to reduce both high density lipoprotein cholesterol levels and increased levels of triglycerides. Acute withdrawal of β-blockade has been associated with an increase in coronary events in patients with hypertension. Finally, recent data from drug rotation studies have suggested that β-blockade may increase central pulse pressure via an increase in ventricular pressure wave reflection from the periphery and a decrease in heart rate. Such effects may be of physiological significance as they have been shown to produce an increase in brain natriuretic peptide (BNP). β-blockade may, therefore, not be the ideal therapy for patients with isolated systolic hypertension and angina as early wave reflection will shift the reflected wave into systole, allowing less time for coronary artery filling during diastole.

Due to individual patient characteristics, β-blockade will have varying degrees of benefit and adverse effects in different patients. The clinician must, therefore, balance the benefits and risks of these drugs in each individual in the clinical setting.

6.12 What is the evidence base for their use?

β-blockers are as effective in the prevention of long term angina symptoms as any of the other classes of anti-anginal agent clinically available. Indeed, a number of studies have suggested greater benefit in terms of symptomatic relief of angina than that seen in patients on monotherapy with other agents.[6] In addition to symptomatic relief, the evidence that β-blockade reduces CHD mortality and morbidity is strong, both in patients post myocardial infarction and in individuals taking β-blockers for other indications. Evidence as to the tolerability of β-blockade relative to the other agents such as nitrates and calcium channel blockers is less secure, although a recent meta-analysis suggested fewer adverse events in patients with stable angina on β-blockade.[7]

6.13 Are there differences between drugs in this class?

A variety of β-blockers are clinically available. There is no consistent body of evidence demonstrating better clinical outcome with one drug compared to another. Therefore, the choice of β-blocker will be influenced by differences in properties within a class. However, care should be taken in ascribing clinical value to basic pharmacological differences between drugs which may lead to only minor clinical differences.

A number of differences exist within the class of β-blockers. These include lipid solubility, route of elimination, β_1 selectivity, and intrinsic sympathomimetic activity. Differences in lipid solubility primarily affect metabolism. Lipophilic β-blockers are metabolised predominantly by the liver and have a relatively short half-life. Highly lipophilic β-blockers were, therefore, originally administered twice or more per day although better formations now allow lipophilic β-blockers to be taken once a day. β-blockers with short half-lives may be more likely to precipitate acute coronary syndromes if withdrawn abruptly in patients with CHD.

Although β-blockers have been classified as possessing or lacking selectivity for cardiac β_1 receptors, such cardioselectivity is relative and diminishes at doses that are commonly used in clinical practice.

CALCIUM CHANNEL BLOCKERS

6.14 What is their mechanism of action?

Calcium channel antagonists inhibit calcium entry to cells via voltage dependent and slow recovery channels. These agents are essentially classified by the type of calcium channel they inhibit and by their binding site. There are two important voltage dependent calcium channels: the

L type (which is long acting) and the T type (or transient channel). The majority of calcium channel blockers clinically available target the L channels and these drugs can be further divided into three classes according to their physicochemical properties and binding sites:

■ *Dihydropyridines* include amlodipine, nifedipine, isradipine, felodipine and nicardipine. These agents all bind to the N binding site.
■ *Benzothiazepines* such as diltiazem bind to the D binding site
■ *Phenylalkylines* such as verapamil bind to the V binding site.

Calcium channel blockers exert three major effects on the cardiovascular system:

■ Vasodilatation via smooth muscle relaxation in both the peripheral and coronary vasculature
■ A negative inotropic effect via an effect on cardiac myocytes
■ A decrease in automaticity and conduction velocity via an effect on slowing of calcium channel recovery in sinus and atrioventricular nodal cells.

The major effects of calcium channel blockers are confined to cardiac and smooth muscle cells. Verapamil mainly affects the heart whereas the majority of dihydropyridines exert a greater effect on vascular smooth muscle. Diltiazem appears to have activity between the two. These actions are beneficial in patients with angina as they reduce myocardial oxygen consumption and, via coronary vasodilatation, increase myocardial oxygen supply.

6.15 What are the indications for their use?

Calcium channel blockers are useful and effective in patients unable to tolerate β-blockade due to coexisting illness (e.g. asthma). In addition to their use in CHD, calcium channel blockers are useful in the treatment of hypertension and supraventricular arrhythmias (verapamil). In addition, calcium channel blockers have been used in patients with primary pulmonary hypertension but with little success. In the treatment of angina, calcium channel blockers have two major indications:

■ in the treatment of stable angina due to fixed coronary artery narrowing
■ in the treatment of vasospasm induced angina.

Calcium channel blockers are particularly effective in the treatment of vasospastic (Prinzmetal's, or variant) angina. This condition often occurs in the absence of fixed arteriosclerotic coronary artery disease; it can occur at rest and is associated with ST segment elevation. All three major classes of calcium channel blocker are equally effective in this condition. The use of calcium channel blockers post myocardial infarction is controversial although diltiazem has demonstrated benefit in non Q-wave myocardial infarction.

6.16 What are the contraindications to their use?

Calcium channel blockers should be used with caution in a number of patient groups. Due to their vasodilator action, patients with low baseline blood pressure may develop hypotension. Patients with poor left ventricular systolic function may be subject to worsening of heart failure due to the negative inotropic effect of calcium channel blockade. However, when these drugs have been evaluated in heart failure they appear to have a neutral effect. Patients with sick sinus syndrome or atrioventricular nodal block may exhibit worsening bradycardia, and calcium channel blockade should be avoided in this group. Calcium channel blockers are absolutely contraindicated in arrhythmias such as Wolff–Parkinson–White syndrome which involve antegrade conduction via an abnormal bypass tract. Severe aortic stenosis is also a contraindication to the use of dihydropyridine calcium channel blockers. Observational studies suggest that the use of short acting calcium channel blockers such as nifedipine may increase cardiovascular morbidity and mortality in patients with unstable angina or post myocardial infarction. In the light of available evidence and the lack of data from prospective randomised trials, it is reasonable to avoid short acting calcium channel blockers in patients with CHD.

6.17 What are their adverse effects?

 As discussed above, short acting calcium channel blockers, especially nifedipine, have been shown to increase myocardial infarction in patients with hypertension[8] and in patients with unstable angina and post myocardial infarction.[9] Treatment with calcium channel blockers, especially the dihydropyridines, may paradoxically exacerbate anginal symptoms. This may be due either to reflex tachycardia increasing myocardial oxygen demand or to coronary steal due to dilatation of coronary arteries that are not actually stenotic and which may decrease myocardial oxygen supply. Combination therapy with a β-blocker may avoid this situation.

Side-effects common across the class of calcium channel blockers include headache, facial flushing, dizziness and ankle oedema. Ankle oedema and flushing are, however, more common with dihydropyridine therapy. Gastrointestinal adverse effects include nausea, oesophageal reflux and especially verapamil constipation. Rare side-effects are gingival hyperplasia and cataracts.

6.18 What is the evidence base for their use?

A large body of evidence supports the benefit of calcium channel blockade in terms of reducing the frequency of anginal attacks, increasing the time to angina during exercise, and exercise duration in addition to increasing the time to demonstrable ischaemia. Two large trials – Total Ischaemic Burden European Trial (TIBET) and Angina Prognosis Study in Stockholm (APSIS) – have addressed the issue of calcium channel blockers in stable angina; both compared calcium channel blockade to that with a β-blocker. In the TIBET study 608 patients were followed for 1 year, receiving either slow release nifedipine or atenolol. The two regimens were equally efficacious although withdrawal was more common in patients taking nifedipine. The APSIS study compared long term treatment with verapamil or metoprolol in patients with stable angina. Both drugs had similar effects on mortality, cardiovascular endpoints and quality of life. Although conflicting, the overall evidence also supports the use of calcium channel blockers in patients with silent myocardial ischaemia.

6.19 Are there differences between drugs in this class?

Although dihydropyridines, verapamil and diltiazem are all calcium channel blockers, there are important differences between these agents in terms of both their pharmacologic and adverse effect profile. For example, nifedipine, diltiazem and verapamil bind to overlapping sites on the L type channel and show different affinities for the different physiological states of the channel, in that verapamil and diltiazem but not nifedipine bind preferentially to the channel in its inactivated state. This leads to preferential blockade of L type channels by verapamil and diltiazem in which the channel undergoes negative cycling through its inactivated state. This may explain the effect of these compounds on pacemaker cells.

The dihydropyridine nifedipine has a greater effect on vascular smooth muscle than on cardiac myocytes or conduction cells. In contrast, the non-dihydropyridines have greater degrees of negative inotropic, chronotropic and dromotropic effects and, because of reflex tachycardia, dihydropyridines are more likely to precipitate rate-dependent angina than the non-dihydropyridines.

NITRATES

6.20 What is their mechanism of action?

Organic nitrates act by relaxing smooth muscle. In common with inorganic nitrates such as sodium nitroprusside, they increase cyclic guanosine monophosphate (cGMP) formation via activation of soluble cytosolic guanylate cyclase and this is the basis of their cellular effect. Unlike inorganic nitrates, organic nitrates such as GTN and isosorbide dinitrate need to be enzymatically converted to nitric oxide (NO) in order to produce smooth muscle relaxation and vasodilatation. This conversion is known to involve a reaction with tissue –SH groups. NO – either alone or after forming a reactive nitrosothiol intermediate – then activates soluble guanylate cyclase and increases cGMP formation. The exact mechanism by which a rise in cGMP causes relaxation is still unclear but it may involve activation of protein kinases which oppose the increased levels of calcium caused by contractile agonists; alternatively it may affect a number of cellular pathways directly.

The anti-anginal effects of organic nitrates are multifactorial. The release of NO induces vasodilatation in both arteries and veins. At low doses the major effect of nitrates is venodilatation but higher doses also produce arteriolar dilatation. At doses commonly used in clinical practice, nitrates dilate epicardial coronary arteries. However, venodilatation results in venous pooling which reduces both left and right heart filling pressures, leading to decreased cardiac preload and a reduced cardiac output. Coupled with dilatation of the large epicardial arteries, there is an increase in total coronary subendocardial flow. Nitrates also reduce wave reflection in the arterial tree, which results in a reduction in left ventricular workload. Dilatation of peripheral resistance arteries (seen at higher doses) may also result in a decreased systemic arterial pressure. In normal subjects GTN increases coronary flow despite a decrease in mean arterial pressure. Since both arterial pressure and cardiac output are reduced, myocardial oxygen demand is reduced, and this, coupled with increased coronary blood flow, results in an increase in the oxygen content of coronary sinus blood. GTN has also been shown to divert blood from normal to ischaemic areas of the myocardium via a mechanism thought to involve collateral vessel dilatation.

In summary, nitrates reduce myocardial oxygen consumption by decreasing arterial pressure and cardiac output. In addition, they redistribute coronary blood flow to ischaemic areas. However, it should be borne in mind that many patients develop tolerance to nitrates, especially if long acting drugs are used continuously. The mechanisms involved in the generation of nitrate tolerance are not as yet fully understood although depletion of free sulphydryl groups may be involved. Tolerance to the anti-anginal effects of short acting drugs such as GTN does not occur clinically.

Finally, nitrates inhibit platelet aggregation, a mechanism which may be useful, especially in unstable angina.

6.21 What are the indications for their use?

Short acting nitrates such as GTN are used most commonly to treat acute episodes of angina. A single 0.4 mg tablet of GTN administered sublingually will usually abort an anginal attack within 2–5 minutes. Sublingual GTN is also used in the short term prophylaxis of angina. A patient with stable angina about to undertake activity likely to provoke an attack of angina may find that prophylactic use of GTN may permit physical activity without any anginal symptoms. For the treatment of chronic stable angina, isosorbide mono- and dinitrate are commonly used in clinical practice as prophylaxis against angina. It is important to ensure a nitrate-free window during the day (asymmetrical dosing) or use a once-a-day modified release preparation (with a built-in nitrate-free period) to prevent tolerance.

6.22 What are the contraindications to their use?

A major contraindication to the use of nitrates is the presence of aortic stenosis or hypertrophic cardiomyopathy. In such patients with significant disease, a decrease in ventricular preload caused by nitrate administration may acutely depress cardiac output and lead to refractory hypotension, even in patients with normal resting blood pressure. In addition, another contraindication to the use of nitrates is the phenomenon of nitrate resistance. In contrast to patients with nitrate tolerance, in which persistent exposure to organic nitrates results in a decreased effect, nitrate resistance is unexplained and results in a primary lack of response to nitrates. The mechanisms involved are unclear but the phenomenon is more common in subjects with diabetes, suggesting some degree of overlap with insulin resistance since GTN and insulin produce similar haemodynamic effects.

6.23 What are their adverse effects?

 The most common adverse effect of organic nitrates is headache due to cerebral arterial vasodilatation. It is most frequently associated with rapid administration of higher doses of GTN. The major drawback of long term nitrate therapy is the development of tolerance. This can be avoided by ensuring nitrate-free periods of 8–12 hours per day. In addition to headache, patients may experience flushing and occasionally tachycardia. Dilatation of peripheral resistance arteries may also result in a decrease in systemic arterial pressure, an effect than can paradoxically provoke angina if coronary perfusion is impaired since this is mostly dependent on diastolic blood pressure.

6.24 What is the evidence base for their use?

Oral nitrates are effective in the long term prevention of anginal symptoms when used as a sustained release preparation. Both isosorbide mono- and dinitrate are effective in controlling symptomatic angina in placebo-controlled trials. The evidence base for nitrate patches is less strong and trial results have been conflicting. In addition, they are considerably more expensive than oral therapy. High dose patches are more effective than low dose provided there is a suitable patch-free interval.

6.25 Are there differences between drugs in this class?

The major differences between drugs in the nitrate class are due to onset and duration of action and first pass metabolism in the liver. GTN is a rapid, short acting nitrate whereas isosorbide mono- and dinitrate are longer acting. Isosorbide dinitrate undergoes extensive first pass hepatic metabolism whereas isosorbide mononitrate does not. The sustained release preparation of isosorbide mononitrate can be given once daily at doses between 30 and 240 mg.

6.26 Do nitrates interact with sildenafil?

Sildenafil is a phosphodiesterase 5 inhibitor which inhibits the breakdown of cGMP, thus prolonging and potentiating the action of nitric oxide. Therefore, the combination of sildenafil with nitrates can lead to severe hypotension. This may be clinically important as impotence is often associated with CHD and, therefore, there is substantial likelihood that patients with angina may be taking both nitrates and sildenafil. If so, this should not be encouraged without specialist medical advice and monitoring. However, the interaction between sildenafil and nitrates may not necessarily always be disadvantageous. Indeed, recent small studies suggest that in patients with refractory hypertension, the addition of sildenafil to nitrates may allow for better blood pressure control, especially in patients with isolated systolic hypertension.

POTASSIUM CHANNEL OPENERS

6.27 What is their mechanism of action?

Adenosine triphosphate (ATP)-sensitive potassium channels (K_{ATP}) were originally described in animal cardiac myocytes. K_{ATP} channels are present in the heart and vasculature and play an important role in the modulation of cardiovascular function. On opening, potassium channels cause an increased efflux of potassium ions from the cell resulting in a negative shift of the arresting membrane potential causing hyperpolarisation. This in turn leads to an inhibition of calcium influx or indirect calcium antagonism. These events result in a fall in intracellular calcium concentrations producing relaxation of vascular smooth muscle and vasodilatation. Currently nicorandil is the only clinically available potassium channel opener with an anti-anginal effect. It confers benefit via a dual action of potassium channel opening combined with a nitrate-like effect.

6.28 What are the indications for their use?

Nicorandil is indicated for the prevention and long term treatment of angina and is available in the UK in 10 and 20 mg doses. Since nicorandil has been shown to mimic ischaemic preconditioning, it has been suggested that it may possess cardioprotective properties. However, the clinical value of such properties remains to be established.

The benefits of nicorandil have recently been assessed in the Impact of Nicorandil in Angina (IONA) study. This randomised study examined the effect of nicorandil versus placebo in 5126 patients with stable angina. There was a significant reduction in coronary events in the treatment group.[10] In addition, two recent studies support the use of nicorandil in unstable angina and myocardial infarction. Interestingly, unlike nitrates, tolerance to the effects of nicorandil has not been reported.

6.29 What are the contraindications to their use?

Contraindications to the use of nicorandil would include those of nitrates (*see Q. 6.22*). In addition, the use of nicorandil in patients taking oral hypoglycaemic drugs, which act via inhibiting potassium channel opening, is a potential contraindication. Whether the interaction between nicorandil and such agents is clinically important is currently unclear. Care should also be taken in administering nicorandil to patients taking phosphodiesterase 5 inhibitors (e.g. sildenafil) for impotence (*see Q. 6.26*).

6.30 What are their adverse effects?

 The occurrence of headache is common but is usually of a transitory nature. It can be reduced by using lower doses initially and then progressive upward titration. Flushing is less common than with nitrates but, similar to nitrates, hypotension and tachycardia can occur.

ASPIRIN

Aspirin was originally isolated from the bark of the willow tree and has a simple chemical structure. It is readily absorbed from the gut and is usually administered at an initial dose of 300 mg and given as a maintenance dose of 75–300 mg daily. Aspirin exerts its beneficial therapeutic effects through its antiplatelet effects. Inhibition of prostaglandin synthesis and, in particular thromboxane A_2 production, causes a reduction in platelet stimulation and aggregation. This has the consequence of reducing intravascular thrombus formation and prevents vascular occlusion.

The plasma half-life of aspirin is 1–2 hours but, because of its irreversible inhibition of the cyclo-oxygenase enzyme, its duration of action is maintained for the lifetime of the platelet (*see Fig. 10.1*). Restoration of normal platelet function, therefore, requires the generation of new platelets.

6.31 What are the indications for its use?

Aspirin, or acetyl salicylic acid, is a simple but very effective treatment for all patients with coronary heart disease and cardiovascular disease in general (*Box 6.4, see also Fig. 6.2*). Aspirin is currently indicated for the primary, secondary and emergency treatment of patients with coronary heart disease.

6.32 What are the contraindications to its use?

Aspirin therapy is contraindicated in patients with an aspirin allergy. A proper history should be obtained as allergic reactions are often over-reported and may not represent a true allergy. This is particularly important where a potentially life-saving treatment, such as aspirin, is involved. In patients with a clear history of facial swelling and laryngeal oedema, aspirin should not be administered. In the absence of severe symptoms and where doubt exists, rechallenging the patient may be appropriate. Aspirin (and other non-steroidal agents) should be avoided in patients with a clear history of aspirin-induced asthma.

There are several relative contraindications that reflect the adverse effects of aspirin. The decision to use aspirin depends upon the relative risk and benefits of therapy. The major hazards of aspirin treatment relate to an increased risk of bleeding complications or gastric ulceration. Patients at increased risk of bleeding include those with peptic ulcer disease, history of gastrointestinal haemorrhage, intracranial haemorrhage, concomitant oral anticoagulants and uncontrolled hypertension. In patients undergoing surgery, aspirin should be withdrawn 5–7 days before surgery if the risks of bleeding are unacceptably high. However, where possible, patients with cardiovascular disease should remain on aspirin in the perioperative period

---

BOX 6.4 Indications for aspirin use
- Acute or prior myocardial infarction
- Stable or unstable angina
- Coronary artery bypass surgery or percutaneous coronary intervention
- Prevention in higher risk patients without cardiovascular disease
- Peripheral vascular or cerebrovascular disease
- Non-valvular atrial fibrillation
- Prophylaxis of venous thromboembolism

as this will reduce perioperative cardiovascular complications and events. Care should be taken when administering aspirin to people taking other non-steroidal anti-inflammatory drugs because this increases the risk of gastrointestinal problems and may lessen the benefit of aspirin.

6.33 What are its adverse effects?

 As with all effective antiplatelet agents, there is a small but significant increased risk of bleeding associated with aspirin use.

Aspirin use is associated with ~0.2% risk of intracranial haemorrhage and ~0.6% risk of major gastrointestinal haemorrhage over 10 years. This risk appears to be independent of the cardiovascular risk. Therefore, for primary prevention, aspirin should be considered in those patients with a significant risk of developing cardiovascular disease. The United States Preventative Services Task Force has estimated that for 1000 patients with a 5% risk for CHD events over 5 years, aspirin would prevent 6–20 myocardial infarctions but would cause 0–2 haemorrhagic strokes and 2–4 major gastrointestinal bleeding events. For patients with a risk of 1% over 5 years, aspirin would prevent 1–4 myocardial infarctions but would still cause 0–2 haemorrhagic strokes and 2–4 major gastrointestinal bleeding events.

Gastrointestinal bleeding may also occur as a consequence of gastric irritation and the inhibition of protective mucosal prostaglandins. This risk appears to be dose related and is higher when ≥300 mg daily is given. Enteric coatings do not appear to meaningfully alter this risk, despite considerably increasing cost, but reducing the dose to a maintenance of 75 mg daily would appear to ensure efficacy while lowering the bleeding risk.

In occasional patients, aspirin can exacerbate asthma. Again, the risks and benefits should be considered but the vast majority of patients with asthma are able to tolerate aspirin well and should not be denied the preventative benefits of aspirin in the presence of concomitant cardiovascular disease.

6.34 What is the evidence base for its use?

There have been many randomised controlled trials of aspirin use in cardiovascular disease. This evidence base is substantial and the benefits incontrovertible in the context of CHD.[2]

The Antiplatelet Trialists' Collaboration[2] performed the definitive meta-analysis of aspirin use in approximately 100 000 patients and reported a 25% (95% confidence intervals (CI), 21–29%) relative reduction in the future risk of cardiovascular events (combined endpoint of death, myocardial infarction and stroke). In particular, the incidence of non-fatal myocardial infarction was reduced by 34% (95% CI, 28–40%).

These benefits have also been consistently demonstrated in the setting of acute coronary syndromes where the outcome is even more dramatic. Acute aspirin therapy reduces the event rate by 30–50% in patients with unstable angina or acute myocardial infarction.

OTHER ANTIPLATELET AGENTS

6.35 What other agents are available?

Aspirin is a relatively weak antiplatelet agent and this has encouraged the development of more effective antiplatelet drugs. There are three main classes of antiplatelet agent in addition to aspirin: dipyridamole, thienopyridines and glycoprotein IIb/IIIa receptor antagonists (*see Fig. 10.1*).

DIPYRIDAMOLE

Dipyridamole is both a vasodilator and antiplatelet agent. It acts through inhibition of platelet phosphodiesterase and thereby blocks cAMP conversion to adenosine triphosphate. This leads to inhibition of platelet adhesion, aggregation and lengthening of shortened platelet survival time.

THIENOPYRIDINES

There are two main agents in this class: ticlopidine and clopidogrel. They antagonise the adenosine diphosphate (ADP) receptor of the platelet and thereby inhibit platelet aggregation. Other agonists can stimulate platelets through alternative pathways, such as thromboxane A_2, but thienopyridines are able to block the amplification process whereby ADP released from platelets causes further platelet activation and aggregation (*see also Q. 10.6*).

The administration and pharmacodynamics of clopidogrel are very similar to aspirin. It can be given as a 300 mg oral bolus with a daily maintenance dose of 75 mg. Clopidogrel has a very short plasma half-life and is rapidly metabolised by the liver to a carboxylic acid derivative. Clopidogrel itself is a prodrug and requires conversion by cytochrome P_{450} to an active thiol derivative that irreversibly modifies the ADP receptor. Thus, restoration of normal platelet function requires the generation of new platelets.

GLYCOPROTEIN IIB/IIIA RECEPTOR ANTAGONISTS

The glycoprotein IIb/IIIa receptor is the final common pathway through which platelets aggregate. Therefore, whatever the stimulus, these agents will prevent platelet aggregation. However, they do not inhibit platelet activation and degranulation.

There are several different types of glycoprotein IIb/IIIa receptor antagonist that fall into three broad categories: antibodies, small peptides or non-peptidic oral agents.

■ *Abciximab* is a murine human chimeric monoclonal antibody that blocks the receptor and can only be administered parenterally.

- *Eptifibatide* and *tirofiban* are also parenteral agents that are small-molecule peptides. Eptifibatide was designed from barbourin, a disintegrin, and contains an analogue sequence of fibrinogen that blocks fibrinogen binding to the glycoprotein IIb/IIIa receptor. Tirofiban was designed to inhibit the RGD peptide sequence in a manner specific to fibrinogen.
- *Sibrafiban* is an orally active non-peptidic glycoprotein IIb/IIIa receptor antagonist that has been administered as long term secondary prevention in patients with an acute coronary syndrome.

6.36 What is the evidence base for their use?

DIPYRIDAMOLE

The Antiplatelet Trialists' Collaboration has clearly established that dipyridamole does not have any role in the prevention or treatment of CHD.

There is some evidence from a single large trial, the European Stroke Prevention Study 2, that combination dipyridamole and aspirin therapy may have a role in cerebrovascular disease.[11] In meta-analyses, dipyridamole plus aspirin reduced vascular events but not deaths when compared to aspirin alone in patients presenting with a recent cerebrovascular event. However, this positive finding is entirely attributable to the influence of the results of the European Stroke Prevention Study 2.

THIENOPYRIDINES

In comparison to placebo, ticlopidine has been shown to reduce cardiovascular events by between 26 and 51% in patients with an acute stroke or coronary syndrome. However, this evidence was preceded and superseded by trials demonstrating similar efficacy with aspirin. Therefore, aspirin remains the first line agent of choice in these conditions.

The CAPRIE trial[12] was a head-to-head comparison between clopidogrel and aspirin in nearly 20 000 patients with vascular disease. The study population was composed of approximately three equal sized populations of patients with coronary heart disease, cerebrovascular disease and peripheral vascular disease. There was a statistical, but very small clinical, benefit in favour of clopidogrel in terms of reducing cardiovascular events over a 3-year follow-up period (relative risk reduction 8.7%; 95% CI, 0.3–16.5%, $p = 0.043$). For many clinicians, the CAPRIE trial demonstrated, at least, the equivalence of aspirin and clopidogrel therapy in the secondary prevention of cardiovascular disease. Given the limited additional benefit, clopidogrel remains a second line agent for the secondary prevention of CHD.

The CURE trial[13] assessed whether the combination of aspirin and clopidogrel was superior to aspirin alone in the immediate and short term (3–12 months) treatment of patients with unstable angina or non-ST segment elevation myocardial infarction. This study was able to demonstrate a 20% relative risk reduction in the combined endpoint of cardiovascular death, stroke and myocardial infarction. This benefit appeared to be predominantly driven by a reduction in re-infarction and recurrent severe myocardial ischaemia.

Whether the combination of clopidogrel and aspirin is superior to aspirin alone in the prevention of CHD remains to be established, but is the subject of ongoing studies such as the CHARISMA trial.

GLYCOPROTEIN IIB/IIIA RECEPTOR ANTAGONISTS

There are several agents that block the glycoprotein IIb/IIIa receptor. These agents are diverse in their chemical structure and pharmacokinetics. Much has been made of their differing pharmacology and pharmacodynamics.

Glycoprotein IIb/IIIa receptor antagonists may reduce the endpoints of death, myocardial infarction and recurrent ischaemia by ~10% in patients with acute coronary syndromes. This benefit is of borderline significance and does not appear to be sustained in the long term. In contrast, in patients undergoing percutaneous coronary intervention, these agents produce a sustained reduction in death, myocardial infarction or recurrent revascularisation by 20–30%.

Several studies have suggested that there are important differences between the agents used: some agents are more beneficial in patients with unstable angina while others benefit patients undergoing percutaneous coronary angiography. In either event, these agents have a limited benefit in patients with acute coronary syndromes, are unlikely to help those patients who do not undergo percutaneous coronary intervention, and have unknown benefits in those patients already receiving clopidogrel.

In terms of secondary prevention, glycoprotein IIb/IIIa receptor antagonists appear to be as equally efficacious as aspirin in the secondary prevention of CHD. However, in contrast to clopidogrel, glycoprotein IIb/IIIa receptor antagonists appear to increase mortality in patients with CHD already receiving aspirin therapy and, therefore, have no role in the secondary prevention of CHD in these patients.

In summary, the use of glycoprotein IIb/IIIa receptor antagonists appears to be limited to the cardiac catheterisation laboratory and specifically in those patients with an acute coronary syndrome who are at particularly high risk and are likely to undergo percutaneous coronary intervention.

6.37 What are their adverse effects?

Dipyridamole
Dipyridamole may cause gastrointestinal upset, flushing and rashes. However, it is usually well tolerated. Dipyridamole does potentiate the

action of intravenous adenosine and the latter should be administered at half the usual dose.

Thienopyridines

The first thienopyridine, ticlopidine, had a small (2–4%) but significant risk of potentially fatal agranulocytosis. Its use was, therefore, limited to patients with severe adverse aspirin reactions or short term combination therapy such as following intracoronary stent implantation. Long term therapy required regular haematological surveillance. Subsequently, clopidogrel was developed as an analogue of ticlopidine. Clopidogrel does not have demonstrable bone marrow toxicity and has excellent long term tolerability.

As with all antiplatelet agents, there is an increased bleeding risk with clopidogrel alone, but particularly in combination with aspirin. In the CURE trial,[13] major bleeding was increased by 34% and minor bleeding by 78% in patients receiving clopidogrel plus aspirin in comparison to those receiving aspirin alone.

Unlike aspirin, clopidogrel does not increase the incidence of peptic ulcer disease. However, in the presence of gastrointestinal haemorrhage, bleeding will be increased by clopidogrel therapy.

Glycoprotein IIb/IIIa receptor antagonists

These agents produce potent inhibition of platelets through blockade of the glycoprotein IIb/IIIa receptor: the final common pathway of platelet aggregation. However, they do not inhibit platelet activation and degranulation and may potentially increase platelet activation.

To inhibit platelet aggregation and thrombus formation, there must be over 80% inhibition of the platelet glycoprotein IIb/IIIa receptors. If inhibition falls below this threshold, intense platelet aggregation may occur. This may explain the apparent paradoxical increase in mortality with the secondary prevention trials of long term glycoprotein IIb/IIIa receptor antagonism in combination with aspirin.

Bleeding risk is increased with glycoprotein IIb/IIIa receptor antagonism. Given that these agents are often used during percutaneous coronary intervention, vascular complications are also increased, especially when continuous intravenous heparin therapy is administered after the procedure. There is also a risk of developing thrombocytopenia, especially with abciximab, although this is usually self-limiting.

OTHER ANTI-ANGINAL DRUGS

6.38 Do antioxidants improve angina?

Epidemiological evidence suggests that antioxidants may have a number of beneficial effects on CHD, including slowing the progression of angiographically proven coronary atheroma and preventing restenosis post angioplasty. Supplementation with antioxidants improves endothelial function and enhances the beneficial effect of statins on coronary endothelial function and vasomotion. Vitamin C has also been shown to attenuate abnormal vasoreactivity in 32 patients with coronary vasospastic angina.[14] However, direct evidence concerning morbidity or mortality benefits of antioxidants is limited. The CHAOS study demonstrated that oral supplementation with vitamin E significantly decreased non-fatal myocardial infarction in patients with angiographically proven coronary heart disease.[15] A further small study of coenzyme Q10 demonstrated improved exercise tolerance and time to angina in patients with chronic stable angina.[16] However, the Heart Protection Study failed to find any benefit from antioxidant supplementation and a study involving 1795 male Finnish smokers with angina showed no benefit of either vitamin E or β-carotene. Therefore, in terms of outcome there appears to be no benefit of antioxidant vitamin supplementation even in high risk patients with CHD (*Fig. 6.5*).[17]

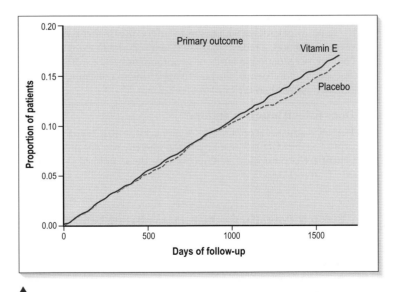

▲

Fig. 6.5 Lack of benefit of vitamin E supplementation. Kaplan–Meier estimates of the effect of vitamin E on the composite outcome of non-fatal myocardial infarction, stroke or death from cardiovascular causes; p = 0.3. (From Yusuf et al.[17] Copyright © 2000 Massachusetts Medical Society. All rights reserved.)

In terms of dietary supplementation, L-arginine has been shown to improve abnormal endothelial function and a recent small study showed improvement of exercise capacity and quality of life in patients with stable angina receiving dietary supplementation with a medical food bar enriched with L-arginine.[18]

6.39 Does cholesterol reduction improve angina?

The large statin-based, cholesterol reduction trials clearly demonstrate that statins appear to have benefits beyond cholesterol reduction alone, in both patients with established CHD and those at high risk of developing it. This may be due to a number of mechanisms including improving coronary endothelial function and stabilisation of atheromatous coronary artery plaque. The benefits of cholesterol reduction in acute coronary syndromes have recently been evaluated in four randomised controlled trials.[19] Three studies showed a benefit from early initiation of statin therapy, whereas one trial showed neither benefit nor harm. However, all trials to date have lacked the power and design to sufficiently evaluate whether cholesterol reduction reduces mortality and re-infarction in patients with acute coronary syndrome. Therefore, a further four ongoing trials have been designed with sufficient power to address this important question.[19]

In terms of patients with coronary artery disease that is not amenable to revascularisation, a recent small study showed benefit from aggressive cholesterol reduction in terms of symptoms and echocardiographic assessment of ischaemia, the benefit appearing to reflect improved vascular function rather than the burden of atheroma.[20]

6.40 Does fish oil improve angina?

Fish oil is a rich source of omega-3 fatty acids, which have been shown to protect against CHD. The mechanisms whereby fish oils produce clinical benefit are as yet unclear, but may include those outlined in *Box 6.5*.

BOX 6.5 Potential mechanisms mediating benefits of fish oil supplementation

- Anti-arrhythmic effect
- Anti-inflammatory effect
- Antithrombotic effect
- Improvement of endothelial function
- Hypotensive effect
- Decreased triglycerides
- Plaque stabilisation

Death from CHD was reduced by 32.5% in the Diet and Reinfarction Trial (DART)[21] and by 29.7% in the more recent GISSI-Prevenzione trial.[22] In the latter, the majority of benefit in terms of decreased mortality was due to a reduction in sudden death, suggesting an anti-arrhythmic effect.

A small study has suggested that dietary supplementation with fish oil can produce symptomatic improvement in angina. However, a study involving 3114 men with angina demonstrated that those given fish oil capsules had a higher risk of cardiac death than individuals not given advice to eat oily fish.[23] One recent study has shown that individuals with a polymorphism of the 5-lipoxygenase gene may receive greater benefit from fish oil consumption.[24]

Apparently there is evidence to support the use of fish oil supplementation post myocardial infarction (GISSI study) and recent American Heart Association guidelines support fish oil supplementation in patients with documented CHD.[25] A large double-blind randomised placebo-controlled trial (SO.FOL.OM) is currently evaluating the benefits of fish oil supplementation in subjects with coronary and cerebral atherosclerosis.

To date no trials have examined the potential benefit of fish oil in primary prevention and future trials may help to identify patients who could benefit most from fish oil supplementation, such as those with stable angina or multiple cardiovascular risk factors.

 PATIENT QUESTIONS

6.41   Should everybody take aspirin?

Although it has recently been advocated that everyone over the age of 55 should take aspirin, this has not yet been shown to be beneficial. However, the benefits of aspirin in patients who already have coronary heart disease have been clearly demonstrated and all such individuals should take aspirin. Again, aspirin given acutely at the time of a heart attack is also beneficial and is now part of standard medical practice. In addition, patients who have had coronary artery bypass surgery should receive aspirin as should those who have had balloon angioplasty. Since subjects with diabetes have a greatly increased risk, they should probably all be treated with aspirin unless there is a compelling reason not to do so.

Recently aspirin has been shown to be beneficial in individuals without coronary heart disease but who also have additional risk factors such as high blood pressure or high levels of cholesterol. The recommended dose would be 75 mg per day in such individuals. Care should be taken in patients with high blood pressure and this should be well controlled in subjects taking aspirin.

Coronary revascularisation for angina

7

7.1　What types of coronary revascularisation are available?

Coronary revascularisation refers to techniques that attempt to improve the flow of blood to the heart. The two main methods of coronary revascularisation are percutaneous coronary intervention (PCI) and coronary artery bypass surgery (CABG). These approaches are discussed below.

There are other novel forms of revascularisation that are under development but are yet to be established in routine clinical practice. These include transmural laser revascularisation (TMR) and angioneogenesis.

■ *Transmural laser revascularisation*: TMR has been assessed in patients with severe angina that is uncontrolled on medical therapy and is not amenable to PCI or CABG. The technique uses an argon laser to produce channels through the myocardium that are in continuity with the left ventricular cavity. This can be performed percutaneously or through a thoracotomy. It was developed to improve myocardial perfusion by permitting the flow of blood from the left ventricular cavity into the channels and thence the myocardium. However, the channels created by the laser rapidly thrombose and might not improve blood flow per se. Some workers have suggested that TMR may exert beneficial effects through the disruption of myocardial neuronal pain pathways. The true clinical benefits of TMR have been questioned and its clinical efficacy has not been widely accepted.

■ *Angioneogenesis*: Areas of ischaemic myocardium often cause the opening of collateral vessels to improve perfusion. This has led some investigators to develop techniques that may encourage this process and lead to new vessel formation: so-called angioneogenesis. The approach has been to administer angiogenic factors, or adenoviral vectors containing genes encoding for these factors, to stimulate new vessel growth. These angiogenic factors include vascular endothelial growth factor and fibroblast growth factor. They can be administered by direct intramyocardial injection or coronary perfusion. The utility of this technique has yet to be established but is currently being evaluated in patients with severe angina that is uncontrolled on medical therapy and is not amenable to PCI or CABG.

PERCUTANEOUS CORONARY INTERVENTION

7.2　What is percutaneous coronary intervention?

Percutaneous coronary intervention (PCI) refers to mechanical procedures that are carried out at the time of coronary angiography. This principally involves the use of percutaneous transluminal coronary angioplasty (PTCA) and stent implantation.

PTCA seeks to restore blood flow to ischaemic myocardium by transiently inflating a balloon in a coronary stenosis and thereby increasing the luminal area of the artery. To maximise and maintain dilatation of the vessel after PTCA, an intracoronary stent (a coated metallic 'scaffolding') is implanted within the artery (*Fig. 7.1A*). Several additional techniques that may also be used to help in this process are discussed in more detail in *Box 7.1*.

In patients with acute coronary syndromes, large amounts of thrombus may be present in the vascular lumen. PTCA can cause embolisation of the clot and impair tissue perfusion. Under such circumstances, thrombectomy devices can be used to extract thrombus from the artery and facilitate subsequent PCI (*Fig. 7.2*).

PCI in saphenous vein bypass grafts does pose some particular problems. The atheromatous tissue that forms in such grafts is often very friable and can cause distal embolisation. Special devices can now be deployed at the end of the graft that act as a net to catch the large debris generated during PTCA.

7.3 How is PCI performed?

The PTCA procedure is performed in a catheter laboratory using the same radiological equipment as for coronary angiography. Anxious patients may be offered simple benzodiazepine sedatives prior to the procedure. A haemostatic sheath is inserted through the skin into a peripheral artery under local anaesthesia. Fine hollow coronary catheters are manipulated, under fluoroscopic guidance, into the coronary ostium via this peripheral sheath. Several views of each coronary artery are taken, each requiring the hand injection of 5–10 mL of contrast agent.

Once the lesion has been identified, intravenous heparin is administered. A guide catheter is inserted and the coronary artery engaged. A guide wire is passed along the catheter and threaded down the coronary artery until the tip of the wire is positioned in the lumen of the distal vessel. The angioplasty balloon is then threaded over the guide wire and advanced up the catheter and down into the artery. Using the balloon markers in combination with contrast injections, the balloon is positioned such that the stenosis is at its midpoint. The balloon is then inflated to 4–6 atmospheres of pressure. During the inflation process, balloon expansion is monitored using fluoroscopic screening to ensure adequate expansion of the stenosis. The balloon is left inflated for variable lengths of time; typically 10–90 s. Following deflation, the balloon is withdrawn into the guide catheter before assessment of the PTCA site is then made to confirm a satisfactory result.

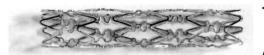

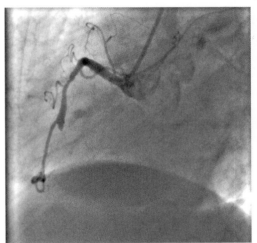

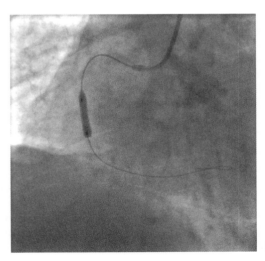

Fig. 7.1 A, A coronary artery stent; **B**, an occluded coronary artery; **C**, inflated angioplasty balloon.

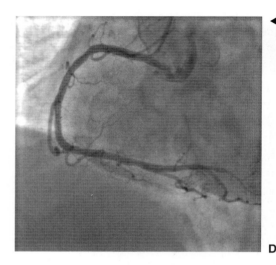

◀ **Fig. 7.1 cont'd**
D, the same artery after PTCA and deployment of a stent.

D

BOX 7.1 Adjuvant techniques for PTCA

PTCA may be unsuccessful or fail when the coronary atheroma is bulky, and especially when it is heavily calcified. Atherectomy devices can be used under these circumstances to enable successful intervention to be performed:

■ *Directional atherectomy* uses a modified angioplasty balloon that contains a chamber and cutting piston. Here the balloon is inflated and the atheroma prolapses into the chamber where it is excised by the cutting piston.

■ *Rotational atherectomy*, or rotablation, is more widely used and employs a small diamond studded burr that is rotated at 160–180 000 rpm and 'sands' down the calcified atheroma. It produces such small fine debris that it does not cause distal embolisation and vessel occlusion.

Both approaches can occasionally cause vessel perforation.

A stent is usually implanted at the angioplasty site. This is performed using a similar technique to angioplasty. The stent comes premounted on an angioplasty balloon. It is inserted into the coronary artery in the same way as a balloon and is implanted into the artery wall by inflation of the angioplasty balloon to high pressures (8–12 atmospheres). Deflation and removal of the balloon leaves the implanted stent deployed in the artery (*see Fig. 7.1*).

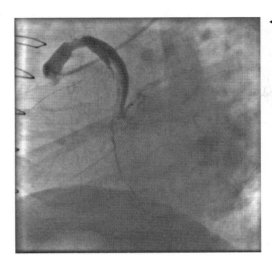

Fig. 7.2 Angiogram showing a massive thrombus in a saphenous vein graft of a patient presenting with an acute coronary syndrome.

7.4 Who should undergo PCI?

The potential risks and benefits of coronary revascularisation need to be evaluated by both patient and physician. Factors such as coronary anatomy, comorbidity and patient preference will have a major bearing on the appropriateness and type of revascularisation procedure undertaken. Moreover, in young patients it is appropriate to consider intervention for both prognostic and symptomatic reasons whereas among elderly patients improving quality of life is likely to be the main aim of therapy.

In patients with chronic stable angina, PCI is generally considered when there has been a failure of medical therapy to control or treat symptoms. It should also be considered in those patients who have unacceptable side-effects from anti-anginal drug therapy. PCI is particularly suited to single-vessel coronary artery disease but it may also be an acceptable alternative to CABG in some patients with multivessel disease. CABG may be a more appropriate form of revascularisation than PCI and should be considered particularly in patients with severe patterns of coronary artery disease such as left main stem stenosis and severe proximal triple-vessel disease (*Box 7.2*).

Coronary angiography with a view to PCI should be considered in most patients with an acute coronary syndrome, especially where there are clinical or biochemical markers of an adverse prognosis such as the development of pulmonary oedema, extensive electrocardiographic changes or a rise in cardiac troponin.

BOX 7.2 Indications for percutaneous coronary intervention

Stable angina

Patients with limiting angina despite optimal medical therapy who:

- would benefit symptomatically from PCI
- have single- or two-vessel disease
- have previously undergone CABG (an initial strategy of PCI is preferable to repeat CABG)
- have multivessel disease and are unsuitable for CABG, but have a suitable severe stenosis – 'culprit lesion PCI'.

Unstable angina

Patients with:

- unstable angina and markers of high cardiovascular risk
- persistent crescendo or unstable angina despite optimal medical therapy.

Myocardial infarction

- Primary angioplasty
- 'Rescue' angioplasty is sometimes considered in those patients who have presented early and have failed to reperfuse with thrombolytic therapy
- Limiting post myocardial infarction angina despite optimal medical therapy

---

PCI is the treatment of choice for acute ST-segment elevation myocardial infarction. When used early, it is associated with a 30% reduction in mortality compared to patients treated with thrombolytic therapy (*Fig. 7.3*).[1] It may also be considered in patients who have failed to reperfuse with thrombolytic therapy: so-called 'rescue angioplasty'. There is little evidence base for this approach and, where it is to be employed, it is best used early.

7.5 When should coronary stents be used?

There is an extensive evidence base for intracoronary stent implantation. The use of intracoronary stents has dramatically reduced the complication and recurrence rate associated with PTCA.

Balloon angioplasty often causes arterial dissection and occasionally vessel occlusion. Stent implantation is a very effective way of treating dissections by tacking down the intimal flap against the artery wall. This restores vessel patency and prevents acute vessel closure. Previously, this may have necessitated emergency bypass surgery. Since the introduction of intracoronary stenting, emergency CABG is a rare outcome of PCI.

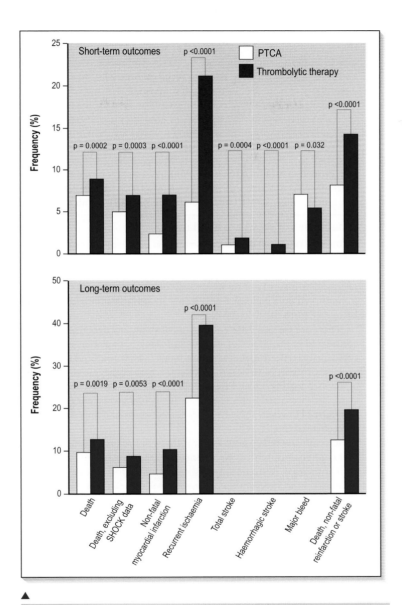

Fig. 7.3 Effect of percutaneous transluminal coronary angioplasty (PTCA) on mortality. Short and long term clinical outcomes in individuals treated with primary PTCA or thrombolytic therapy. (From Keeley et al.[1] Reprinted with permission from Elsevier.)

Intracoronary stent implantation is not only an effective means of treating dissections and to 'bail out' acute vessel closure, but is also of benefit in most patients undergoing PTCA. Immediately following PTCA, there is a tendency for the vessel to recoil and the gains made by the angioplasty may be lost. In the medium term, PTCA may also be complicated by a proliferative response to the barotrauma imparted to the muscular arterial wall. This response is known as neointimal hyperplasia and causes restenosis at the site of angioplasty. The restenosis rate after PTCA alone is around 25–40%. Intracoronary stent implantation reduces vascular recoil but does not prevent neointimal hyperplasia. Thus, the restenosis rate is reduced but not abolished by stent implantation and currently runs at 10–20%. In-stent restenosis is more likely in smaller vessels (≤2.5 mm), longer stents, bifurcation lesions or patients with diabetes mellitus.

7.6 What types of stent are available?

Stents are composed of metallic struts that are formed from a solid metallic cylinder or produced by wire coiling (*see Fig. 7.1A*). Certain metals, such as nickel containing alloys, can cause problems for those patients with a nickel allergy. The majority of stents are balloon expandable and come premounted on a balloon. Some stents are self-expanding and are deployed by release from the delivery device.

There are various different designs of stent. Features that need to be considered in the choice of stent include length, diameter, radial strength, cell density (reflecting the degree of metal framework) and flexibility.

Coated stents have become available where agents are impregnated into a polymer coating. One of the first to be employed was a heparin-coated stent. This was used to try to reduce the incidence of stent thrombosis and restenosis. However, these heparin-coated stents had limited benefits above 'bare metal stents'.

Recently, there has been major interest in the use of drug eluting stents that contain antiproliferative agents. Sirolimus is a macrolide antibiotic with antifungal, immunosuppressive and antimitotic properties that has been used in the prevention of renal transplant rejection. Sirolimus coated stents are associated with a dramatic reduction in the incidence of in-stent restenosis, with failure of target vessel revascularisation falling from 21.0 to 8.6% in the SIRUS study of 1058 patients with coronary heart disease (*Fig. 7.4*).[2] Paclitaxel is a microtubule-stabilizing agent with potent antitumour activity that has also been successfully used in stent coatings with similar reductions in in-stent restenosis.

7.7 What is the role of glycoprotein IIb/IIIa antagonists?

The glycoprotein IIb/IIIa receptor is the final common pathway through which platelets aggregate. These agents cause potent inhibition of platelet

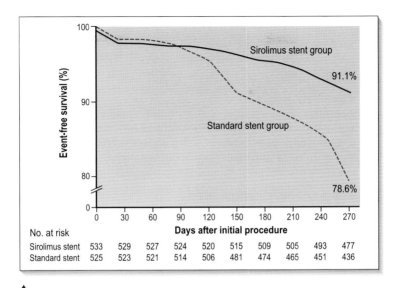

Fig. 7.4 The rate of event-free survival was significantly higher in the sirolimus stent group than in the standard stent group (p <0.001). (From Moses et al.[2] Copyright © 2003 Massachusetts Medical Society. All rights reserved.)

aggregation and have particular utility when used during PCI (*see Qs 6.35–6.37*).

There are several different types of glycoprotein IIb/IIIa receptor antagonist. Abciximab, eptifibatide and tirofiban are all parenteral agents that can be used as adjunctive therapy in patients undergoing PCI. They appear to be equally efficacious in the reduction of major adverse cardiovascular events (cardiovascular death, non-fatal myocardial infarction and target vessel revascularisation) although one trial suggested that 30-day but not 6-month outcome was better with abciximab than with tirofiban.

Glycoprotein IIb/IIIa receptor antagonists have significant benefits in patients undergoing elective PCI as well as those requiring urgent procedures for an acute coronary syndrome. They appear to be of particular benefit where the procedure is in a high risk individual with intracoronary thrombus in situ.

Bleeding risks are increased with glycoprotein IIb/IIIa receptor antagonism. Vascular complications are more common, especially when continuous intravenous heparin therapy is administered after the procedure. Therefore, it is routine practice to remove the arterial sheath before recommencing heparin therapy should it be required.

7.8   What are the benefits of PCI?

Immediate angiographic success is achieved in approximately 95% of PCI procedures, and this is usually mirrored by clinical success with alleviation of anginal symptoms.

CHRONIC STABLE ANGINA

Compared with medical treatment, PTCA is associated with significantly less angina for at least 2 years after the procedure.[3,4] This reduction in anginal symptoms is associated with a diminished requirement for anti-anginal drug therapy, an increase in exercise capacity and an overall improvement in quality of life.

ACUTE CORONARY SYNDROMES

An initial strategy of coronary angiography and revascularisation in all patients admitted with unstable angina or non-ST segment myocardial infarction reduces the risk of death, myocardial infarction or recurrent severe ischaemia. How much of the mortality benefit is due to PCI rather than CABG is unknown but both revascularisation strategies do appear to reduce recurrent myocardial ischaemia.

Patients with an acute ST segment elevation myocardial infarction have improved survival, less recurrent infarction and fewer strokes when treated with PCI rather than intravenous thrombolytic agents. This is particularly prominent for recurrent infarction with a relative risk reduction of 65% (95% confidence intervals (CI), 55–73%). These benefits were seen in both the short (4–6 weeks) and longer term (6–18 months).

Patients with an acute coronary syndrome who subsequently develop recurrent symptoms despite medical therapy gain a marked improvement in symptoms and angina following PCI.

7.9   What are the risks of PCI?

Percutaneous coronary intervention is associated with several important complications. There are those risks associated with cardiac catheterisation itself such as peripheral arterial dissection, bleeding and embolisation. The commonest problem is a haematoma or false aneurysm at the site of arterial puncture. This risk is increased during PCI because of the extensive use of heparin and antiplatelet agents. False aneurysms or persistent bleeding may require prolonged compression, injection or surgical repair.[5]

Percutaneous coronary intervention in elective procedures has resulted in angiographic success rates of 96–99%, with Q-wave myocardial infarction rates of 1–3%, emergency coronary bypass surgery rates of 0.2–3%, and unadjusted in-hospital mortality rates of 0.5–1.4%. In diabetic patients, the 5-year cardiac mortality was 7.5%.[6]

The immediate procedural risks of PCI predominantly relate to technical complications from angioplasty and stent insertion. These include coronary arterial dissection, vessel occlusion, coronary perforation, embolisation and 'no reflow phenomenon'. The last arises due to vessel spasm and embolisation where, despite a patent proximal vessel, there is no blood flow down the coronary artery. These complications can cause myocardial infarction, hypotension, tamponade, arrhythmias and ultimately death. Elective PCI is a relatively safe procedure with less than 0.5% mortality.

The short and long term complications usually relate to stent thrombosis or restenosis. Stent thrombosis is unusual (~1%) but is more likely to occur with inadequate antiplatelet therapy or suboptimal stent deployment. In-stent restenosis occurs in 10–20% of patients and is predominantly due to neointimal hyperplasia. It is usually manifest by 3–6 months after the procedure. This complication is likely to be reduced by the introduction of drug eluting stents.

7.10 What treatment should be given after the procedure?

After PCI, all patients should receive intensive antiplatelet therapy. Evidence supports the use of the combination of aspirin and clopidogrel. Many centres use aspirin 300 mg and clopidogrel 75 mg once daily for 1 month before reverting to aspirin alone at 75–300 mg daily. The duration of intensive antiplatelet therapy needs to be prolonged in patients who have a drug eluting stent implanted because of the delayed re-endothelialisation associated with the antiproliferative coatings. Current recommendations suggest at least 2 months of combination clopidogrel and aspirin therapy. However, recent evidence from the CREDO trial[7] suggests that, in patients who are to undergo PCI, pretreatment with clopidogrel at least 6 hours before the procedure and continued for up to 1 year after the procedure may be of benefit.

All patients should continue to receive standard secondary prevention therapy for coronary heart disease (CHD).

CORONARY ARTERY BYPASS GRAFT SURGERY

7.11 What is coronary artery bypass graft surgery?

Coronary artery bypass graft (CABG) surgery is a technique where either venous or arterial conduits are used literally to 'bypass' fixed proximal coronary stenoses by the creation of anastomoses from the aorta to the distal coronary arteries. This improves myocardial blood flow and tissue perfusion, and is a very effective method of relieving angina and myocardial ischaemia. The technique is challenging and requires a large surgical team including the support of a 'perfusionist', a dedicated anaesthetic team and a cardiothoracic intensive care unit.

7.12 How is CABG performed?

Coronary artery bypass grafting is performed as an open surgical procedure under general anaesthesia. Access to the heart is achieved with a midline sternotomy incision. Cardioplegia is administered to arrest the heart, with the functions of the heart and lungs being assumed by a pump and oxygenator: cardiopulmonary bypass. Saphenous veins, harvested from the legs, are grafted from the aorta to the distal coronary arteries beyond the occlusive lesions. Both internal mammary arteries may be utilised and other arteries including the gastroepiploic, inferior epigastric or radial arteries may be used as grafts.

On completion of the surgery, the chest is closed with sternal wire sutures and the patient transferred for observation on the cardiothoracic intensive care unit. In uncomplicated procedures, the patient is rapidly weaned off the ventilator and allowed to regain consciousness. For some patients, prolonged ventilation and support from inotropes or intra-aortic balloon pump may be required, especially where there is significant left ventricular impairment or complex surgery.

A period of cardiac rehabilitation is often necessary to facilitate healing and encourage the return of normal activities.

7.13 Who should undergo CABG?

Coronary artery bypass graft surgery is an appropriate intervention in patients with limiting angina despite optimal medical treatment who have suitable coronary anatomy, i.e. symptomatic patients with:

- a significant left main stem stenosis of ≥50%
- triple-vessel disease
- two-vessel disease including a significant proximal left anterior descending (LAD) artery stenosis.

Intervention is especially useful if left ventricular function is impaired or the exercise test is strongly positive.

Coronary artery bypass graft surgery may also be considered for patients with ischaemic symptoms other than angina. For example, CABG may be appropriate in patients with severe heart failure due to reversible ischaemic myocardial dysfunction. It may also be employed in those individuals where myocardial ischaemia provokes life-threatening malignant arrhythmias.

Coronary artery bypass graft surgery is also undertaken in patients who are undergoing valvular surgery. This may be undertaken even in the absence of anginal or other ischaemic symptoms.

7.14 Which type of grafts should be used?

As a consequence of graft vasculopathy, saphenous vein bypass grafts have an accelerated failure rate which is particularly evident beyond the fifth year. Therefore, arterial conduits are being increasingly employed in an attempt to improve graft survival. The internal mammary arteries are the principal conduits to have been assessed although other conduits, such as the radial and gastroepiploic arteries, may also be used.

At 10 years following CABG, 83% of internal mammary artery grafts remain patent compared with only 41% with saphenous vein grafts. Observational and quasi-experimental studies have shown that this improved patency rate is associated with better long term survival and a reduction in the risk of angina, hospitalisation, myocardial infarction and reoperation. Overall, patients who undergo CABG only with saphenous vein grafts have a 1.6 times greater risk of death over 10 years compared with those receiving an internal mammary artery graft. There is now an increasing attempt to use exclusively arterial grafts, so-called 'total arterial revascularisation (TAR)', when undertaking CABG rather than using saphenous vein grafts.

7.15 What is 'off-pump' surgery?

Cardiopulmonary bypass is associated with a significant incidence of complications that include neurological sequelae such as memory loss and stroke. Techniques have been developed whereby grafting can be undertaken without the need for cardiopulmonary bypass: so-called 'off-pump' surgery. Whether this approach reduces neurological sequelae has yet to be definitively established.

The attachment of grafts to a beating and constantly moving heart creates a challenge for the surgeon. However, various methods have been used to assist this technically demanding approach, including the use of a platform and fixation stage that is able to minimise the motion of the arterial segment of interest, thereby assisting the grafting process.

7.16 Does CABG require a sternotomy?

A midline sternotomy is the primary surgical approach to achieve access to the heart and undertake bypass grafting. However, this causes significant morbidity in the immediate and longer term postoperative period. In order to avoid the necessity of a sternotomy, surgeons can perform minimally invasive surgery where several small 2–4 cm incisions are made and, using thoracoscopic techniques, graft surgery can be performed. This has many advantages including faster recovery times and shorter hospital stays. However, this is not possible in all patients.

7.17 What are the symptomatic benefits of CABG?

In comparison to medical therapy, CABG significantly improves symptoms of angina, exercise capacity and reduces the need for anti-anginal therapy. Following CABG, three-quarters of patients are free of angina at 1 year and a half at 5 years. Moreover, patients experience a better quality of life and report less limitation in physical activity, with nearly three-quarters of patients returning to work within 1 year.

7.18 What are the survival benefits of CABG?

In comparison to medical therapy, CABG improves long term (10 year) survival in patients with stable angina, and in particular those with more than 50% left main stem stenosis. Survival benefits are also seen in patients with triple- or two-vessel disease including proximal stenosis of the LAD coronary artery. However, patients with two-vessel disease excluding proximal LAD stenosis or single-vessel disease do not derive any survival advantage from CABG. Patients with abnormal left ventricular function or strongly positive exercise tests derive greater absolute survival benefit from CABG than from medical therapy.

The survival benefit for coronary artery surgery is, therefore, related to the severity of coronary artery disease. Those with the most severe coronary artery disease have the most to gain from coronary artery surgery and the benefits are greatest in those with left main stem disease followed by triple-vessel disease and least for those with single- or two-vessel disease.

7.19 What are the risks of CABG?

Coronary artery bypass grafting is a safe operation with elective surgical mortality frequently reported at around 2–4%, depending on the case mix. Various factors influence surgical mortality including age, sex, the degree of left ventricular impairment and the presence of other comorbid conditions including diabetes mellitus, obesity and hypertension. Other complications of CABG include myocardial infarction, stroke, infection and haemorrhage. However, for many patients, wound healing and discomfort are the major limiting problems in the first months after surgery.

PCI OR CABG

7.20 Which type of coronary revascularisation improves symptoms best?

There is a significant difference in the reported symptoms of angina when comparing the two main forms of coronary revascularisation. The prevalence of angina at 1 year after revascularisation is considerably higher in patients treated with PCI (1.5–2-fold) but at 3 years this difference is significantly attenuated and is not detectable. Reflecting these differences in efficacy, 18% of patients treated by PCI require additional revascularisation in the form of CABG within 1 year while in subsequent years the requirement for CABG is around 2% per year. Overall, at 5 years, the need for subsequent revascularisation procedures is 8% in patients treated with CABG and 54% for PCI. These differences may have been overestimated because of the technical improvements in PCI made in recent years. This has recently been demonstrated in the Stent or Surgery (SoS) trial although there remain significant differences in the need for recurrent revascularisation with 6% of those patients treated by CABG requiring repeat procedures compared to 21% for those undergoing PCI.[8]

7.21 Which type of coronary revascularisation improves prognosis best?

A meta-analysis of eight large randomised trials comparing PCI ($n = 1710$) with CABG ($n = 1661$) over a mean follow-up of 2.7 years has shown no significant difference in prognosis between the two revascularisation strategies.[9] The BARI trial[10] was published after the Pocock meta-analysis and is the largest study comparing PCI and CABG ($n = 1829$). This also showed no significant difference in survival or risk of myocardial infarction between PCI and CABG.

This similarity does not mean that the two forms of coronary revascularisation are equivalent. These trials and meta-analysis did not assess whether PCI was non-inferior or superior to CABG. PCI for stable CHD has never been shown to improve prognosis and indeed is associated with an increased cardiovascular event rate. Therefore, only CABG can truly be demonstrated to be associated with an improved prognosis. Moreover, in the recent SoS trial of patients with multivessel disease, PCI was associated with a higher mortality (5%) when compared to CABG (2%).

The Duke database ($n = 9263$) suggests that patients with single-vessel disease, or two-vessel disease without involvement of the proximal LAD artery, have better clinical outcomes with PCI than with CABG. This contrasts with the findings of the Pocock meta-analysis where the combined endpoint of death or myocardial infarction in single-vessel disease appeared to be less with CABG than with PTCA (4.5% versus 7.2%). However, this subgroup analysis encompassed only three trials with small numbers ($n = 350$ for each group) and the authors question the reliability of this finding. Moreover, in contrast to the Duke database, the patients in these randomised trials were highly selected populations: for example, the RITA-1 trial recruited only 3% of patients undergoing an angiogram.

7.22 Which factors predict benefit?

The prognostic and symptomatic benefits of coronary revascularisation are driven by the completeness and success of the revascularisation process itself. This is determined by coronary anatomy. Some patients may present with diffuse disease that affects the entire length of the vessel. This pattern of disease is often seen in patients with diabetes mellitus. Under such circumstances, it may not be technically feasible to perform conventional coronary revascularisation with either PCI or CABG. The stenoses may not be amenable to dilatation or bypass, or the distal vessels have poor run off. For some patients, coronary revascularisation is offered speculatively in the belief that their anginal symptoms may improve while recognising that the procedure may fail to achieve this.

The outcome from PCI is determined by the nature and type of lesion. It has been recognised that certain plaque types are associated with more complications and a worse outcome. The American Heart Association classification (*Box 7.3*) outlines three main lesion types although the type B lesion has subsequently been divided into types B1 and B2. Type A lesions are associated with a high (92%) success and a low (2%) complication rate. In contrast, the more complex lesions have success and complication rates of 61 and 21% respectively.

The prognostic benefits of CABG are determined principally by the coronary anatomy and left ventricular function. Patients with severe left main stem stenosis will gain a mean survival benefit of 19 months (95% CI, 6–33 months), those with triple-vessel disease 6 months (95% CI, 2–9 months) and those with impaired left ventricular function 11 months (95% CI, 5–17 months). Patients with severe angina (Canadian Cardiovascular Society grades III and IV) or an abnormal exercise tolerance test also gain benefit from surgery with an increase in survival of 7 months (95% CI, 3–12 months) and 5 months (95% CI, 2–8 months) respectively.

7.23 How is the type of revascularisation procedure chosen?

Selection of the appropriateness and the type of revascularisation procedure will be heavily influenced by technical aspects of the coronary anatomy, patient's age, patient preference and the local waiting times for the revascularisation procedures.

BOX 7.3 American Heart Association classification of coronary stenoses for percutaneous coronary intervention

Type A lesions (high success, >85%; low risk)
- Discrete (<10 mm length)
- Concentric
- Readily accessible
- Non-angulated segment, <45°
- Smooth contour
- Little or no calcification
- Less than totally occlusive
- Not ostial in location
- No major branch involvement
- Absence of thrombus

Type B lesions (moderate success, 60–85%; moderate risk)
- Tubular (10–20 mm length)
- Eccentric
- Moderate tortuosity of proximal segment
- Moderately angulated segment, >45°/<90°
- Irregular contour
- Moderate to heavy calcification
- Total occlusion <3 months old
- Ostial location
- Bifurcation lesions requiring double guide wires
- Some thrombus present

Type C lesions (low success, <60%; high risk)
- Diffuse (>2 cm in length)
- Excessive tortuosity of proximal segment
- Extremely angulated segments >90°
- Total occlusion >3 months old
- Inability to protect major side branches
- Degenerated vein grafts with friable lesions

- *Coronary anatomy*: For some patients, CABG and PCI are not feasible due to the nature of the coronary atheroma such as diffuse, severe and distal disease, whereas patients with discrete and proximal lesions may be appropriate for either PCI or CABG. The coronary anatomy is also an indicator of future risk and prognosis. Patients with significant left main stem disease or triple-vessel coronary artery disease are at particularly high risk and, where appropriate, should be offered coronary revascularisation.

■ *Patient preference*: What is considered a satisfactory level of symptoms, or what is optimal medical therapy, may vary greatly from patient to patient. Those patients with a frustrated and active lifestyle may require intervention at an earlier stage with objectively less severe angina than those with a quiet and sedentary lifestyle.

■ *Comorbidity*: It is also important to appreciate that patients with the greatest perioperative risk may also have the most to gain prognostically from revascularisation and a balance must be met. The presence of an adverse clinical factor is, therefore, not a contraindication to surgery and patients should be assessed on an individual basis.

■ *Procedural*: The major advantages of PCI over CABG surgery are that it usually requires only an overnight inpatient stay, is performed under local anaesthesia, does not require a sternotomy, has a shorter rehabilitation period, incurs a lower procedural cost and can be repeated. Subsequent procedures are as likely to be as successful and uncomplicated as the initial procedure. However, it must be remembered that not all lesions are suitable for PCI. When the main objective of revascularisation is relief of angina it may be advisable to consider PCI of the lesion that is thought to be responsible for the patient's symptoms, even if there is evidence of multivessel disease which might otherwise be treated by CABG. This strategy is often appropriate in symptomatic patients with multivessel coronary artery disease who have a single exceptionally severe stenosis and many minor lesions, or in those patients who are unsuitable for CABG because of comorbid conditions such as cerebrovascular disease or chronic obstructive airways disease. It is also a reasonable option in situations where surgical revascularisation with CABG would be incomplete and may not, therefore, confer prognostic benefit.

■ *Patients with prior CABG*: At 5 years after CABG, 50% of patients will have redeveloped angina and, by 12 years, 30% will have undergone repeat revascularisation. Repeat CABG is associated with a higher risk and a lower likelihood of benefit than the initial intervention. In an analysis of 632 non-randomised patients with previous CABG requiring either elective repeat CABG or PCI, complete revascularisation was achieved in 40% of patients receiving PCI compared to 90% undergoing CABG. However, complications were significantly lower with PCI and survival was similar at 1 year and 6 years of follow-up. Both procedures resulted in similar event-free survival from death, infarction and angina but by 6 years further revascularisation by either repeat PCI or CABG was significantly higher with PCI.

7.24 Can all patients be revascularised?

Coronary revascularisation is not appropriate or feasible in all patients. Patients with single- or two-vessel disease who are asymptomatic do not require coronary revascularisation. Furthermore, such patients do not mandate revascularisation even in the presence of symptoms unless their exercise tolerance, quality of life or lifestyle is limited despite optimal medical therapy.

The pattern of atheroma may preclude conventional coronary revascularisation. As already indicated, the feasibility and success of revascularisation are determined predominantly by the coronary anatomy and lesion type. Diffuse coronary atheroma affecting the distal vessels with poor run off is unattractive for coronary revascularisation. Moreover, some coronary vessels may be occluded and fibrosed with no residual lumen.

7.25 How long does the revascularisation last?

Both forms of coronary revascularisation have a failure rate. PCI may fail early because of acute vessel closure and stent thrombosis. Restenosis at the site of PCI remains a problem but is likely to become less of a problem with drug eluting stents. Restenosis currently runs at 10–20% and predominantly occurs in the first 2–6 months after the procedure. Thereafter, restenosis and recurrence relates to the underlying atherosclerotic process of CHD.

For CABG, there is again an early, intermediate and longer term failure rate for bypass grafts. Early graft failure is, as with PCI, usually related to technical problems at the time of the procedure and arises from graft thrombosis. In saphenous vein grafts, this can be as high as 18% at 30 days post surgery. Subsequent graft failure in the first year is up to 30% and reflects the development of a neointimal hyperplastic response similar to that observed after PCI and stent implantation. In the longer term, graft failure occurs at 2–3% per year, such that at 10 years more than 50% of saphenous vein grafts have occluded. The longer term graft failure arises from the development of graft vasculopathy with atheromatous-type deposits being laid down in the intima of the vein graft. This graft 'atheroma' is friable and has features distinct from those associated with native coronary arteries.

7.26 Which factors influence the effectiveness of coronary revascularisation and reduce the need for repeat procedures?

There are several significant clinical characteristics (*Box 7.4*) that may influence the efficacy and outcome of coronary revascularisation. It is important to appreciate that patients with the greatest perioperative risk may also have the most to gain prognostically from revascularisation and a balance between these concerns must be made. The presence of an adverse factor is, therefore, not a contraindication to surgery and patients should be assessed on an individual basis.

The four biggest predictors of outcome for CABG are age, previous cardiac surgery, peripheral vascular disease and renal failure. Patients who undergo CABG over the age of 75 years have an operative mortality that is five-fold higher than patients who are under 55 years. Previous CABG or the presence of peripheral vascular disease increases the risk by three- to four-fold whereas renal failure is associated with the worst outcome with a greater than five-fold increased risk of death. Other predictors of an adverse outcome include impaired left ventricular function, multivessel disease, diabetes mellitus, female sex and low body surface area.

The effectiveness of PCI is principally driven by lesion type (*see Box 7.3*). However, several other factors also play a role in the outcome from PCI. Vessel diameter is a strong predictor with a poorer outcome, particularly in vessels ≤2.5 mm. The length of artery treated is also an important predictor, with longer lesions having a much higher restenosis rate. In keeping with CABG, clinical factors of advanced age, diabetes mellitus, multivessel disease and impaired left ventricular function are associated with a worse outcome. Patients without diabetes mellitus who are under 60 years with single-vessel disease and good left ventricular function have an excellent prognosis with PCI.

BOX 7.4 Factors influencing the risks and benefits of coronary revascularisation

- Advanced age
- Number of vessels affected
- Female sex
- Severity of angina
- Smoking
- Coexisting valvular disease
- Diabetes mellitus
- Obesity
- Impairment of left ventricular function
- Renal failure
- Cerebrovascular and peripheral vascular disease
- Recent myocardial infarction or episode of unstable angina
- Hypertension
- Chronic obstructive airways disease

7.27 What secondary prevention and lifestyle changes should be considered following coronary revascularisation?

The use of secondary prevention and alterations in lifestyle are particularly important in patients who have undergone coronary revascularisation. The standard approach to secondary prevention in patients with CHD should be applied; however three aspects require particular attention: smoking cessation, antiplatelet therapy and lipid lowering therapy.

- *Smoking cessation* is associated with improved graft and stent patency, lower rates of myocardial infarction and better long term survival in patients undergoing coronary revascularisation. Every effort should be made to encourage smoking cessation.
- *Antiplatelet therapy* is crucial to graft and stent patency. Early combination antiplatelet therapy is essential in coronary stenting and there are some limited data that this may also have a potential therapeutic role in maintaining saphenous vein graft patency. All patients who have undergone coronary revascularisation must be maintained on some form of antiplatelet therapy.
- *Lipid lowering therapy* is equally important in patients who have undergone coronary revascularisation. This is particularly valuable in patients who have undergone saphenous vein bypass surgery. Intensive lipid lowering therapy with high doses of statins is recommended as more marked reductions in plasma low density lipoprotein cholesterol concentrations (<2.6 mmol/L) are associated with improved graft survival and clinical outcomes.

Treatment for unstable angina and non-ST segment elevation myocardial infarction

8

The treatment of unstable angina and non-ST segment elevation myocardial infarction are considered together because the initial management is identical. The distinction between these two diagnoses is made by the subsequent measurements of cardiac markers or enzymes (*see Ch. 3*).

8.1 What are the immediate priorities for management and treatment?

The clinical diagnosis should be established. A detailed clinical history, examination and, where possible, an electrocardiogram performed. Acute myocardial infarction should be suspected if the electrocardiogram shows ST segment elevation of 1 mm or more, or pathologic Q waves in two or more contiguous leads (*see Ch. 9*). Myocardial ischaemia or infarction should also be suspected if there is ST segment depression of 1 mm or more, or T-wave inversion in two or more leads. With a history of prior infarction, comparison with a previous electrocardiogram is essential.

Simple adverse clinical factors include systolic blood pressure below 110 mmHg, bi-basal crepitations and a prior history of coronary heart disease, especially where there is worsening of previously stable angina, a new onset of angina after infarction or after a coronary revascularisation procedure, or pain which is similar to that of a prior myocardial infarction.

All patients with, or suspected as having, an acute coronary syndrome should be admitted to hospital and preferably to a coronary care unit. This requires urgent transfer from the community and an emergency ambulance with paramedic support should be called. The management prior to arrival at hospital is outlined in *Box 8.1*. Once the patient has been admitted to hospital, further management and treatment is as listed in *Box 8.2*.

8.2 Which antiplatelet therapies should be considered and how do they work?

Patients with unstable angina or non-ST segment elevation myocardial infarction should be given aspirin (300 mg stat and 75 mg daily maintenance) and clopidogrel (300 mg stat and 75 mg daily maintenance). High-risk patients should be considered for glycoprotein IIb/IIIa receptor antagonists.

ASPIRIN

Aspirin is a very effective treatment in unstable angina or non-ST segment elevation myocardial infarction. In comparison to placebo, aspirin halves the rate of progression to death, myocardial infarction or stroke. It acts

---

BOX 8.1 Management prior to hospital arrival

■ Intravenous access and electrocardiographic monitoring should be established.

■ In the presence of ongoing pain, opiate analgesia should be administered with an anti-emetic agent (*not* i.m.). When patients are experiencing severe chest pain, there is marked autonomic arousal causing sweating, breathlessness, nausea and anxiety. Opiate analgesia reduces pain and autonomic stimulation. This not only relieves suffering and calms the patient but reduces infarct size and the potential for arrhythmia. Opiate induced emesis increases cardiac work and should be avoided.

■ Oral aspirin (300 mg stat) should be given. In the presence of ischaemia on the electrocardiogram, oral clopidogrel may also be considered (see below).

■ Oxygen therapy should be administered. There is no evidence that this influences outcome but this simple treatment is given in the belief that it may improve oxygenation in watershed areas of myocardial ischaemia.

■ Rapid access to a cardiac defibrillator should be established.

■ Slow release buccal nitrates should be given in the absence of hypotension.

---

through inhibition of the prostaglandin pathways by irreversible blockade of the cyclo-oxygenase pathway. This prevents generation of thromboxane A_2 and reduces platelet aggregation and thrombotic vascular occlusion.

THIENOPYRIDINES

Thienopyridines, such as ticlopidine or clopidogrel (*see Q. 6.35*), have comparable benefits to aspirin in the treatment of patients with an acute coronary syndrome. They act through irreversible inhibition of the platelet adenosine diphosphate receptor. Their use is associated with a halving of the risk of progression to death, myocardial infarction or stroke in patients with unstable angina. In combination with aspirin, clopidogrel causes a further 20% reduction in cardiovascular events in patients with unstable angina or non-ST segment elevation myocardial infarction.[1] Dipyridamole inhibits platelet activation but is of no proven benefit in patients with an acute coronary syndrome.

GLYCOPROTEIN IIB/IIIA RECEPTOR ANTAGONISTS

Glycoprotein IIb/IIIa receptor antagonists block the final common pathway of platelet aggregation to fibrinogen. This causes complete abolition of

---

BOX 8.2 In-hospital management

- History and examination should be performed.
- Electrocardiogram, chest x-ray and blood sampling for full blood count and serum biochemistry including cardiac markers should be undertaken.
- Intravenous access, and electrocardiographic and haemodynamic monitoring should be established.
- Rapid access to a cardiac defibrillator should be established and the patient admitted to a coronary care unit or high dependency area.
- In the presence of ongoing pain, opiate analgesia should be administered with an anti-emetic agent (i.v.).
- Oral aspirin (300 mg stat) and, with electrocardiographic evidence of ischaemia, oral clopidogrel (300 mg stat) should be given (*see Q. 8.2*).
- Oxygen therapy should be administered.
- Fractionated or unfractionated heparin should be given.
- Anti-anginal therapy should be administered. First line therapy should include β-blockade and intravenous nitrates. Where β-blockers are contraindicated (e.g. in patients with asthma), rate limiting calcium antagonists such as verapamil or diltiazem should be given.

---

platelet aggregation and is a potent inhibitor of thrombus formation. Randomised controlled trials have suggested that glycoprotein IIb/IIIa receptor antagonists have a limited role in the treatment of unstable angina and non-ST segment elevation myocardial infarction unless the patient is to undergo percutaneous coronary intervention.[2]

8.3 What is the evidence for benefit?

ASPIRIN

The Antiplatelet Trialists' Collaboration performed the definitive meta-analysis of aspirin use in approximately 100 000 patients and reported a 25% (95% confidence intervals (CI), 21–29%) relative reduction in the future risk of cardiovascular events (combined endpoint of death, myocardial infarction and stroke) (*Fig. 8.1*).[3] In particular, the incidence of non-fatal myocardial infarction was reduced by 34% (95% CI, 28–40%). These benefits have also been consistently demonstrated in the setting of acute coronary syndromes where the outcome is even more dramatic. Acute aspirin therapy reduces the event rate by 30–50% in patients with unstable angina or non-ST segment myocardial infarction.

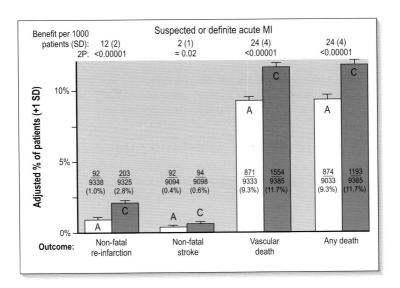

Fig. 8.1 Absolute effects of antiplatelet therapy in patients with an acute myocardial infarction (MI). Data from five trials in patients with acute MI (suspected or definite). A, antiplatelet therapy (mean 1 month); C, control. (From Antiplatelet Trialists' Collaboration,[3] with permission.)

THIENOPYRIDINES

In comparison to placebo, ticlopidine has been shown to reduce cardio-vascular events by between 26 and 51% in patients with an acute coronary syndrome. However, this evidence was preceded and superseded by trials demonstrating similar efficacy with aspirin. The CURE trial ($n = 12\,562$) assessed whether the combination of aspirin and clopidogrel was superior to aspirin alone in the immediate and short term (3–12 months) treatment of patients with unstable angina or non-ST segment elevation myocardial infarction.[1] This study was able to demonstrate a 20% relative risk reduction in the combined endpoint of cardiovascular death, stroke and myocardial infarction. This benefit appeared to be predominantly driven by a reduction in re-infarction (relative risk reduction (RRR) 23%; 95% CI, 11–34%) and recurrent severe myocardial ischaemia (RRR 31%; 95% CI, 9–47%).

GLYCOPROTEIN IIB/IIIA RECEPTOR ANTAGONISTS

Meta-analyses of studies including patients with acute coronary syndromes suggest that glycoprotein IIb/IIIa receptor antagonists reduce the combined endpoints of death and myocardial infarction at 30 days by ~10%.[4] Several studies have suggested that there are important differences between the agents used: some agents are more beneficial in patients with unstable angina while others favour patients undergoing percutaneous coronary angiography. In either event, these agents have a very limited benefit in patients with acute coronary syndromes, are unlikely to help those patients who do not undergo percutaneous coronary intervention, and have unknown benefits in those patients already receiving clopidogrel.

8.4   Which anticoagulants should be used and why?

All patients with unstable angina or non-ST segment elevation myocardial infarction should receive heparin therapy. Meta-analyses indicate that unfractionated heparin reduces the risk of death, myocardial infarction or stroke by a third.

Recently, the role of fractionated heparins has been explored. Fractionated or low molecular weight (LMW) heparins have more selective antithrombin and antifactor Xa activity, and are less likely to induce thrombocytopenia. They also have a more predictable therapeutic range such that LMW heparins can be administered subcutaneously without the need for monitoring the efficacy of anticoagulation. Head-to-head comparisons have demonstrated either similarity or superiority of fractionated heparins. In the ESSENCE trial ($n = 3171$), enoxaparin was associated with a modest 16% relative risk reduction in the primary endpoint of death, myocardial infarction or recurrent angina when compared to unfractionated heparin.[5] While other trials have reported neutral findings, the widespread uptake of LMW heparin use has been driven by its ease of administration and its predictable therapeutic efficacy. The avoidance of making multiple measurements of the activated partial thromboplastin time and adjustments in heparin dose, makes fractionated heparins appealing and potentially more cost effective than unfractionated heparin.

Direct thrombin inhibitors, such as hirudin and lepirudin, have also been assessed in the treatment of patients with acute coronary syndromes. In the GUSTO IIb trial ($n = 12\ 142$), hirudin was compared to unfractionated heparin in patients with an acute coronary syndrome.[6] There was a trend for hirudin to reduce the 30-day event rate of death, myocardial infarction or recurrent ischaemia from 9.8% in those treated with unfractionated heparin to 8.9% (RRR 11%; 95% CI, 0–21%, p = 0.06). Given these modest effects, the widespread use of direct thrombin inhibitors has not been established, particularly given the increasing use of fractionated heparin. However, these agents have a role in patients who cannot receive heparin such as those with heparin-induced thrombocytopenia.

8.5 Should thrombolysis be used?

Thrombolytic therapy is associated with both risks and benefits. The potential devastating effects of stroke, intracranial haemorrhage or gastrointestinal bleeding are major considerations when assessing a patient for thrombolysis.

Meta-analyses of the major thrombolytic trials indicate that, in patients presenting with a history consistent with myocardial ischaemia, intravenous thrombolytic therapy is associated with saving 0 lives per thousand treated in the presence of a normal electrocardiogram, and losing 10 lives per thousand treated with ST segment depression.[7] Therefore, not only is thrombolysis unhelpful, it may actually be harmful, particularly in the presence of ST segment depression.

Thrombolytic therapy has no role in the routine treatment of patients with unstable angina or non-ST segment elevation myocardial infarction.

8.6 Which anti-anginal therapy should be employed?

β-blockers are the first line agents of choice for patients with unstable angina and non-ST segment elevation myocardial infarction. When β-blockers are contraindicated, rate limiting calcium antagonists should be employed. Both these agents reduce the heart rate and have negatively inotropic actions such that they reduce myocardial work and metabolic demands (*see Ch. 6*). These effects are clearly desirable in the context of ongoing myocardial ischaemia and can relieve the symptoms of chest pain.

The addition of intravenous nitrates should be considered in all patients with ongoing chest pain. This should be rapidly up-titrated with close observation of the blood pressure. Nitrates have a complex mode of action including reductions in both afterload and preload as well as direct coronary vasodilator actions. However, continuous infusion of nitrates for 48 hours or more is associated with the development of tolerance (*see Q. 6.20*). Other anti-anginal therapies, such as non-rate limiting calcium antagonists and nicorandil, may also be considered as second line therapy.

8.7 What are the benefits?

SYMPTOMS

All classes of anti-anginal therapy may reduce chest pain in patients with unstable angina or non-ST segment elevation myocardial infarction. They are, therefore, indicated to provide symptomatic relief in these patients.

CLINICAL OUTCOME

There are no contemporary large scale trials of anti-anginal therapy in patients with unstable angina or non-ST segment elevation myocardial infarction. Meta-analyses of previous small trials have suggested that, in patients with unstable angina, β-blockers reduce the rate of progression to myocardial infarction by a modest 13%. However, given their secondary preventative benefits in patients with a recent myocardial infarction, β-blockers should be the first line agent of choice in these patients.

Not all anti-anginal therapies are the same. Non-rate limiting calcium antagonists, such as nifedipine, may cause reflex tachycardia and actually increase cardiac work. This may be undesirable in the context of an acute coronary syndrome and a meta-analysis has suggested that nifedipine may increase event rates in this circumstance.[8]

8.8 Who is at short term risk of recurrent events?

There are several simple clinical markers that identify those patients who are at particularly high risk. Crudely, the number of cardiovascular risk factors is proportional to the future risk. Age is one of the strongest markers of risk. The in-hospital mortality from acute myocardial infarction is ~5% for a 40–50 year old man, rising to more than 30% for an over-75 year old. Other adverse clinical factors include left ventricular impairment, renal failure, other vascular disease, diabetes mellitus, delayed (not within the first 48 hours) ventricular arrhythmias, and pulmonary oedema or haemodynamic compromise at presentation (*Table 8.1*).[9]

There are increasing numbers of biochemical markers that have been associated with an increased risk. These include peak troponin, C-reactive protein and cholesterol concentrations. However, the electrocardiogram remains one of the strongest independent predictors of risk.

8.9 How can I calculate a patient's risk?

A number of risk scoring systems have been developed (*see Q. 3.8*). However, it is important to remember that low risk is not no risk. Patients who have a low risk score still have a significant event rate. For example, a patient with unstable angina without electrocardiographic changes, cardiac marker rise, hypotension or arrhythmia has a 17% chance of re-admission, 9% revascularisation and 2% mortality in the first 6 months.

TABLE 8.1 Predictors of in-hospital mortality for patients with acute coronary syndromes

Variable	OR	95% CI
Admission serum creatinine	1.2	(1.15–1.35)
Heart rate <30/min	1.3	(1.16–1.48)
Systolic blood pressure (per 20 mmHg fall)	1.4	(1.27–1.45)
Cardiac marker rise	1.6	(1.32–2.00)
Age (per 10 years)	1.7	(1.55–1.85)
Killip class	2.0	(1.81–2.29)
ST segment deviation	2.4	(1.90–3.00)
Prehospital cardiac arrest	4.3	(2.80–6.72)

Based on data from Global Registry of Acute Coronary Events (GRACE) dataset,[9] with permission. CI, confidence intervals; OR, odds ratio.

8.10 Who should be considered for coronary angiography and revascularisation?

All patients with unstable angina or non-ST segment elevation myocardial infarction should be considered for coronary angiography and revascularisation, especially where they are at high risk of future cardiovascular events.

There was previous concern that a routine strategy of early invasive intervention with coronary angiography with a view to revascularisation may be associated with an adverse outcome. This was suggested by prior observational studies from the OASIS registry and by the randomised VANQWISH ($n = 920$) trial.[10] However, the latter study was heavily criticised because of the high cross-over rate (~50%) to angiography in the conservative strategy arm of the study. The subsequent FRISC II ($n = 2453$),[11] TACTICS ($n = 2220$)[12] and RITA-3 ($n = 1810$)[13] trials have demonstrated that both high and medium risk patients benefit from a strategy of early invasive investigation with a view to revascularisation.

Selection of patients for angiography is sometimes made using the calculation of the thrombolysis in myocardial infarction (TIMI) risk score (*see Q. 3.8*). This uses seven simple clinical factors to determine the 14-day event rate of patients presenting with unstable angina or non-ST segment elevation myocardial infarction. However, it should be remembered that those patients at highest risk do not necessarily have the most to gain from invasive intervention.

> Post hoc subgroup analysis of the FRISC II study demonstrated that the patients who appeared to benefit most from invasive investigation and revascularisation were male, over 65 years, non-smokers or had a history of prior (>3 months) angina.[11] Ischaemic changes on the electrocardiogram or elevations in cardiac troponins also identified those patients who may benefit from intervention.

8.11 What are the benefits of revascularisation treatment?

SYMPTOMS

Coronary revascularisation in patients with unstable angina or non-ST segment elevation myocardial infarction is associated with a marked reduction in subsequent anginal symptoms and recurrent admission to hospital. In the FRISC II and RITA-3 trials,[11,13] early invasive intervention and revascularisation was associated with a halving of the risk of developing recurrent unstable angina or myocardial ischaemia requiring hospitalisation. The severity of angina and use of anti-anginal therapy are also reduced by 30–50% in the intervention groups.

PROGNOSIS

A strategy of early revascularisation was associated with a significant reduction in mortality in the FRISC II trial: 1-year mortality was reduced by 43%. This is likely to be driven by the surgical revascularisation of patients with left main stem or severe triple-vessel disease.

The prevention of myocardial infarction by revascularisation is controversial. This is because both coronary artery bypass graft surgery and percutaneous coronary intervention are associated with procedural rises in creatine kinase and troponin concentrations. It is, therefore, difficult to classify myocardial infarction because some will be procedural and others spontaneous. This has led some workers to use different definitions for myocardial infarction in those patients undergoing revascularisation. Usually, patients undergoing coronary revascularisation are classified as sustaining a myocardial infarction if the cardiac markers rise more than 1.5–3 times the upper limit of normal whereas for non-revascularised patients the upper limit of normal is used. This inevitably confounds the interpretation of the results since differences are certain to be found if definitions of the endpoint are dependent on the treatment modality. The FRISC II[11] and TACTICS[12] trials used the differing definitions according to treatment allocation and reported a 23 and 33% reduction respectively in the rate of myocardial infarction at 6 months. However, the subsequent RITA-3[13] trial applied the same criteria for myocardial infarction to both treatment groups and found no significant reduction in the rate of myocardial infarction. This is further confused by the fact that the RITA-3 trial used the old WHO definition of myocardial infarction and if the new European Society of Cardiology/American College of Cardiology definition is applied to the RITA-3 trial patients, then there is a highly significant 31–33% reduction in the development of myocardial infarction.

Overall, an early strategy of coronary revascularisation is associated with a significant reduction in morbidity (recurrent myocardial infarction and ischaemia) and mortality.

Treatment of ST segment elevation myocardial infarction

PQ PATIENT QUESTIONS

INITIAL MANAGEMENT

9.1 What are the immediate priorities of management and treatment?

Patients with ST-segment elevation myocardial infarction (*Fig. 9.1*) require early and immediate intervention. To establish the diagnosis, a detailed clinical history, examination and an electrocardiogram should be performed. Acute myocardial infarction should be suspected if the electrocardiogram shows ST segment elevation of 1 mm or more, bundle branch block or pathologic Q waves in two or more contiguous leads.

All patients with, or suspected as having, an acute myocardial infarction should be admitted to hospital, and preferably to a coronary care unit. This requires urgent transfer from the community and an emergency ambulance with paramedic support should be called. Management prior to hospital admission is given in *Box 9.1*. The subsequent management in hospital is outlined in *Box 9.2*.

9.2 Which reperfusion therapies are available?

The treatment of choice for acute ST-segment elevation myocardial infarction is primary angioplasty. Where this is not available, patients should be considered for thrombolytic therapy.

PRIMARY PERCUTANEOUS CORONARY INTERVENTION

In institutions that are able to offer rapid access to a 24-hour catheter laboratory service, percutaneous coronary intervention (PCI) is associated with a greater reduction in mortality and infarct size in comparison to thrombolytic therapy. This is applicable to all patients with acute myocardial infarction, although the widespread use of primary PCI has been limited by the availability of the resources necessary to achieve this highly specialised service. As a consequence, intravenous thrombolytic therapy remains the first line reperfusion treatment in many hospitals.

For some patients, thrombolytic therapy is contraindicated or fails to achieve coronary arterial reperfusion. Early (within 6 hours of symptom onset) emergency PCI may be considered under such circumstances, particularly where there is evidence of cardiogenic shock (*see Q. 9.19*). Clearly, this strategy requires rapid access to the facilities of a cardiac catheterisation laboratory.

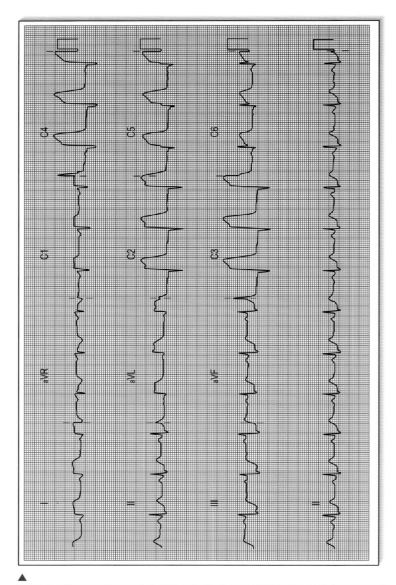

Fig. 9.1 Electrocardiogram of an acute anterior myocardial infarction.

BOX 9.1 Out-of-hospital management of acute myocardial infarction

- Intravenous access and electrocardiographic monitoring should be established.
- In the presence of ongoing pain, intravenous opiate analgesia should be administered with an anti-emetic agent. When patients are experiencing severe chest pain, there is marked autonomic arousal causing sweating, breathlessness, nausea and anxiety. Opiate analgesia reduces pain and autonomic stimulation. This not only relieves suffering and calms the patient but reduces infarct size and the potential for arrhythmia. Opiate-induced emesis increases cardiac work and should be avoided.
- The patient should be considered for pre-hospital thrombolysis, especially where transfer times are substantial. This requires the recording and interpretation of a 12 lead electrocardiogram.
- Oral aspirin (300 mg stat) should be given. There is no requirement for the patient to chew the aspirin or dissolve it into solution.
- Oxygen therapy should be administered. There is no evidence that this influences outcome but this simple treatment is given in the belief that it may improve oxygenation in watershed areas of myocardial ischaemia. It will also assist patients with hypoxia due to acute pulmonary oedema.
- Rapid access to a cardiac defibrillator should be established.

THROMBOLYTIC THERAPY

Thrombolytic agents cause clot dissolution through the activation of plasminogen to plasmin that degrades the fibrin clot and facilitates coronary reperfusion. Many large-scale, randomised, controlled trials have demonstrated the major morbidity and mortality benefits of thrombolytic therapy. However, there are potential risks associated with its use that include fatal intracranial haemorrhage.

The benefit of thrombolytic therapy is time dependent: more rapid administration is associated with greater clinical benefit. There appears to be little benefit from administering thrombolytic therapy beyond 12 hours from the onset of pain: indeed, the frequency of some complications, such as cardiac rupture (*see Q. 9.22*), appears to increase.

BOX 9.2 Hospital management of acute myocardial infarction

- History and examination should be performed.
- Intravenous access, and electrocardiographic and haemodynamic monitoring should be established.
- Rapid access to a cardiac defibrillator should be established and the patient admitted to a coronary care unit or high dependency area.
- Electrocardiogram, chest x-ray and blood sampling for full blood count and serum biochemistry including cardiac markers should be undertaken.
- In the presence of ongoing pain, intravenous opiate analgesia should be administered with an anti-emetic agent.
- Reperfusion therapy should be considered (see below).
- Oral aspirin (300 mg stat) should be given, if not already administered. In patients being considered for primary angioplasty, oral clopidogrel 600 mg stat should be administered.
- Oxygen therapy should be provided.
- Patients should be considered for intravenous β-blockade, particularly in the presence of ongoing pain, hypertension or tachyarrhythmias.

9.3 Should all patients with myocardial infarction be given aspirin?

The ISIS-2 trial (n = 17 187)[1] examined the effects of aspirin, streptokinase and their combination in patients with ST-segment elevation myocardial infarction. This trial demonstrated that both streptokinase and aspirin reduced 30-day mortality and that their combination produced additive benefits.

Unlike thrombolysis, the administration of aspirin therapy is not critically time dependent. It should be administered within the first 12 hours but earlier administration does not mean greater benefit. This is because the beneficial effects of aspirin probably relate to the prevention of re-occlusion of the infarct related artery. Therefore, overvigorous attempts at rapid administration of aspirin are misplaced. There is no need to get the patient to chew the aspirin or dissolve it in water before oral administration.

Aspirin is life saving. Patients who are unconscious should be given aspirin by nasogastric tube. Where oral therapy is contraindicated, intravenous aspirin should be administered. All patients with acute myocardial infarction should receive aspirin therapy. It is only contraindicated in patients with a true aspirin allergy with anaphylaxis.

9.4   What other antiplatelet agents should be administered?

There is no current evidence that other antiplatelet agents reduce mortality in patients with acute ST-segment elevation myocardial infarction.

In patients with acute ST-segment elevation myocardial infarction, it would seem reasonable to use clopidogrel as an alternative to aspirin should a true aspirin allergy with anaphylaxis be present. The potential benefits of adding clopidogrel to aspirin therapy are unknown but clopidogrel should be given to all patients who are to undergo primary angioplasty. There is some evidence that more rapid therapeutic concentrations of clopidogrel can be achieved with an oral dose of 600 mg. Given the known benefits of early pretreatment with clopidogrel in patients undergoing PCI, all patients who are to undergo primary angioplasty should receive oral clopidogrel 600 mg as soon as possible.

Glycoprotein IIb/IIIa receptor antagonists increase the bleeding risk in patients with acute ST-segment elevation myocardial infarction who receive thrombolytic therapy. There have been recent trials to assess whether reduced doses of thrombolysis in combination with abciximab improve outcomes. The GUSTO V ($n = 16\ 588$) trial[2] failed to demonstrate a mortality benefit with abciximab when used in combination with half dose reteplase although there was a small reduction in the rates of re-infarction (2.3% versus 3.5%) and recurrent ischaemia (11.3% versus 12.8%). This modest benefit was associated with a reduced need for urgent revascularisation but at the cost of a doubling in the bleeding risk. In contrast, glycoprotein IIb/IIIa receptor antagonists should be considered early in patients undergoing primary angioplasty or emergency PCI.

Overall, additional antiplatelet agents do not have a role in the routine treatment of patients with acute ST-segment elevation myocardial infarction who have received thrombolytic therapy. For patients undergoing PCI, early oral clopidogrel (600 mg) therapy should be given with the judicious use of intravenous glycoprotein IIb/IIIa receptor antagonists once the angiographic appearances have been established.

THROMBOLYSIS

9.5   Should all patients with myocardial infarction be given thrombolysis?

Not all patients with acute myocardial infarction are suitable or will benefit from thrombolytic therapy. The Fibrinolytic Therapy Trialists' Collaborative Group meta-analysis ($n = 58\ 600$) has demonstrated that only patients with certain electrocardiographic changes benefit from thrombolytic therapy.[3] More widespread use of thrombolysis may be associated with no benefit or indeed harm. The criteria for the administration of thrombolytic therapy are:

- new onset bundle branch block
- ≥ 1 mm ST-segment elevation in at least two contiguous limb leads (I, II, III, aVR, aVL and aVF)
- ≥ 2 mm ST-segment elevation in at least two contiguous chest leads (V_1 to V_6).

The benefits of thrombolysis are very time dependent (*Fig. 9.2*). The major benefit is seen in those patients who are treated within 3 hours of the onset of pain. The mortality benefits continue to be present if treatment is initiated within 12 hours of pain. It can be considered in patients with ongoing or increasing pain who present at 12–24 hours from symptom onset. Once the diagnosis has been established, treatment must be initiated as soon as possible to reduce infarct size and gain the prognostic benefits.

The 35-day mortality benefits of thrombolysis are dependent upon the territory and extent of infarction. Patients presenting with bundle branch block have the most to gain from thrombolysis: 49 lives saved per 1000 treated. Patients with inferior myocardial infarction also gain benefit but to a lesser degree than those with anterior myocardial infarction: 8 and 37 lives saved per 1000 treated respectively. Patients with a normal electrocardiogram or with ST-segment depression should not receive thrombolytic therapy because of the associated adverse outcome: 7 and 14 lives lost per 1000 treated respectively.

9.6 Which thrombolytic agent should be given?

There are three main types of thrombolytic agent: non-specific, clot specific and mutant plasminogen activators. Agents such as streptokinase and urokinase generate plasmin from plasminogen by direct enzymatic activation. This causes rapid breakdown of both fibrin and fibrinogen, and often depletes plasma fibrinogen concentrations.

NON-SPECIFIC AGENTS

Streptokinase is a foreign antigenic protein that is derived from streptococci. In combination with the protein load, intravenous streptokinase administration is associated with a significant incidence of allergic reactions and systemic hypotension. Therefore, its use is not recommended for patients with systemic hypotension or circulatory shock

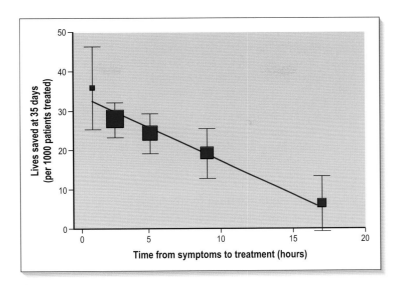

Fig. 9.2 Time dependency of thrombolysis in ST-segment elevation myocardial infarction. (From Fibrinolytic Therapy Trialists' (FTT) Collaborative Group.[3] Reprinted with permission from Elsevier.)

at presentation. Moreover, once it has been administered, there is the potential for the development of neutralising antibodies by the patient. Thus, it is recommended that streptokinase should not be re-administered after 3 days of first administration. The requirement for repeated thrombolysis for re-infarction should then be undertaken with alternative agents, such as tissue plasminogen activator.

CLOT-SPECIFIC AGENTS

Tissue plasminogen activator is released from endothelial cells to induce endogenous fibrinolysis. Some patients with acute ST-segment elevation myocardial infarction have spontaneous reperfusion of the infarct-related artery through this mechanism. However, pharmacological administration of tissue plasminogen activator is able to enhance fibrinolysis and more rapidly establish vessel patency. Tissue plasminogen activator binds to lysine groups on the surface of the fibrin clot and, in the presence of plasminogen, generates plasmin to cause clot dissolution. Because this occurs only at the clot surface, tissue plasminogen activator is clot specific and causes less fibrinogen depletion than streptokinase.

MUTANT PLASMINOGEN ACTIVATORS

Newer mutant tissue plasminogen activators have been developed that have a longer half-life and may have potential improvements in safety and efficacy. Tenecteplase and reteplase are examples of these newer generation plasminogen activators and have the benefit of single or double bolus administration respectively. This assists in the more rapid administration of thrombolytic therapy which is a very important aspect of its clinical application.

Overall, accelerated regimen or mutant tissue plasminogen activators are the thrombolytic agents of choice for acute ST-segment elevation myocardial infarction. However, cost considerations, ease of use and potential adverse effects should be taken into consideration.

9.7 What is the evidence base for their use?

Angiographic substudies of the major thrombolytic trials have suggested that tissue plasminogen activator restores arterial patency more rapidly than streptokinase. Therefore, there was a belief that these benefits in patency rate would be translated into improved clinical outcomes. The ISIS-3 trial[4] ($n = 48 294$) compared the two types of thrombolytic therapy: streptokinase and tissue plasminogen activator. Both agents were associated with a 30-day mortality rate of 10%. There was, however, a small but significant excess of stroke with tissue plasminogen activator (1.39%) compared to streptokinase (1.04%). This was predominantly related to an excess of haemorrhagic stroke.

The GUSTO trial ($n = 41 021$) subsequently looked at several different thrombolytic regimens including the accelerated administration of tissue plasminogen activator over 90 rather than 180 minutes.[5] This trial demonstrated a small but clear 30-day mortality benefit in favour of accelerated tissue plasminogen activator over streptokinase or standard administration of tissue plasminogen activator: a further 10 lives saved per 1000 treated. This is the generally accepted gold standard method of thrombolysis and all subsequent efficacy trials have been made in comparison to this thrombolytic regimen. The mutant tissue plasminogen activator agents have been compared to the accelerated tissue plasminogen activator regimen. Only tenecteplase has been definitively demonstrated to be non-inferior to the accelerated tissue plasminogen activator regimen although reteplase appears to have very similar efficacy. Interestingly, tenecteplase appears to have a lower incidence of haemorrhagic stroke.

9.8 What is the role of heparin in thrombolysis?

There appears to be a rebound prothrombotic effect after the administration of systemic thrombolysis and trials support the use of heparin in the first 48 hours. However, there are differences between the need for anticoagulation with the different types of agent used. All patients treated with tissue plasminogen activator should be anticoagulated with intravenous heparin for the first 48 hours. This is associated with significant reductions in re-infarction rate. In comparison to high dose subcutaneous injection, intravenous heparin use after streptokinase administration does not appear to have any additional benefits, probably because of the associated fibrinogen depletion and derangements in coagulation.

Early open-labelled, randomised trials have indicated that subcutaneous fractionated heparin is as safe and efficacious as intravenous unfractionated heparin following thrombolysis. This provides a simpler mode of heparin administration.

9.9 Can thrombolysis be given outside hospital?

Pre-hospital thrombolysis is a safe and effective treatment for acute ST-segment elevation myocardial infarction. In the GREAT trial ($n = 311$),[6] 3-month mortality was nearly halved when general practitioners in rural Scotland initiated pre-hospital thrombolysis with anistreplase. The time from symptom onset to the administration of thrombolysis was 101 minutes for those receiving pre-hospital thrombolysis and 240 minutes for those treated in-hospital. Clearly, pre-hospital thrombolysis may not be appropriate in an urban setting but it should be considered where transfer times to the hospital are more than 30 minutes.

Pre-hospital thrombolysis does, however, require several important components to make this an effective strategy.

- First, the diagnosis needs to be established. This requires a trained physician or health care professional who can reliably determine the diagnosis from the clinical presentation and the interpretation of a 12 lead electrocardiogram.
- Although performed in the GREAT trial, there is no role for pre-hospital thrombolysis without a diagnostic electrocardiogram because of the risk of inappropriate therapy with potentially catastrophic consequences. Some innovative approaches have included mobile coronary care units or specialist training for ambulance paramedical staff to interpret the electrocardiogram and to administer pre-hospital thrombolysis according to a specific protocol.
- Streptokinase and tissue plasminogen activator are given as continuous intravenous infusions and do not readily lend themselves to rapid administration, especially in a community setting. Single bolus agents, such as anistreplase and tenecteplase, are more appropriate for pre-hospital administration.
- There has been concern with regard to the safety of pre-hospital thrombolysis: in particular the occurrence of reperfusion arrhythmias.

However, this has not been borne out in practice. Randomised controlled trials, particularly in rural areas, have demonstrated the efficacy and practicality of performing pre-hospital thrombolysis. All patients should be transferred by emergency ambulance to hospital with the minimal delay. This should be undertaken with a paramedic crew who are able to undertake electrocardiographic monitoring and to perform cardiac defibrillation.

9.10 Is thrombolysis safe?

Thrombolysis does incur a significant risk of bleeding. This may occur in any region of the body but is most serious when associated with intracranial haemorrhage.

The excess incidence of stroke attributable to thrombolysis is 3.9 per 1000 patients treated. Strokes are more common in the post myocardial infarction period (~1% in the first 35 days) because of embolism from left ventricular mural thrombi. The small excess of stroke caused by thrombolytic therapy is seen only in the first 24 hours and is caused by either intracranial haemorrhage or thromboembolism. The latter occurs in ~50% of cases and is likely to represent thromboembolism from treatment-induced instability of aortic or carotid plaques.

Extracranial bleeding complications occur in patients treated with thrombolytic therapy. Major bleeding, which is life threatening or requires blood transfusion, occurs in 7.3 per 1000 patients treated. These bleeding events are predominantly from gastrointestinal blood loss.

9.11 What are the contraindications to thrombolysis?

The contraindications to thrombolysis predominantly relate to unacceptable increases in bleeding risk (*Box 9.3*). All contraindications should be considered against the potential benefits. In a patient with systemic hypotension and an extensive anterior myocardial infarction, the balance of risk and benefit may favour thrombolytic therapy when the patient has presented 3 weeks after abdominal surgery. The risk to such a patient may be unacceptably high if they had incurred a stroke 2 days previously.

9.12 How can thrombolysis be administered more rapidly, and who should give it?

The necessary immediacy of thrombolytic therapy means that various approaches have been used to shorten the length of time from symptom onset to diagnosis and treatment. Delays in the initiation of thrombolysis

---

BOX 9.3 Contraindications to thrombolysis

Absolute
- Recent haemorrhage, trauma or surgery within 1 month
- Aortic dissection
- Stroke within the past 6 months
- Oesophageal varices and severe liver disease
- Haemorrhagic diathesis
- Acute pancreatitis

Relative
- Menstruation (very low risk)
- Pregnancy
- Uncontrolled hypertension
- Anticoagulant therapy
- Known intracardiac thrombus
- Known abdominal aortic aneurysm

---

are often dominated by the time delay of the patient seeking medical attention. Public health campaigns and initiatives from charities, such as the British Heart Foundation, are now targeted at raising the general population's awareness of the symptoms of myocardial infarction and the need to seek medical attention urgently.

Once the patient has sought medical attention, the delay relates to establishing the diagnosis through the recording of the clinical history, examination and electrocardiogram. Careful attention should be given to the presence of contraindications to thrombolytic therapy. Once the diagnosis of ST-segment elevation myocardial infarction has been made, the physician or attending health care professional should rapidly administer thrombolysis.

There have been various approaches that have been made to improve 'pain-to-needle' and 'door-to-needle' times, as driven by the clinical benefits of more rapid thrombolysis and reinforced by local and national guidelines that set target times for the administration of thrombolysis. Pre-hospital thrombolysis is clearly the best approach to reducing 'pain-to-needle' times and this has been consistently demonstrated in observational and randomised trials. However, this does rely upon adequate training in the interpretation of electrocardiograms by primary health care physicians or paramedical staff. Training and educational programmes have been successfully instituted in the primary care setting and are increasingly being applied nationally. In the pre-hospital setting, tenecteplase appears to be the most appropriate agent to use because of its single bolus administration.

Hospital-based protocol driven 'fast track' systems have been employed to reduce the delay in the administration of thrombolytic therapy. The most successful systems appear to involve the deployment of dedicated nurses who have appropriate expertise and experience of coronary care. The 'fast track' process usually involves consultation with an attending physician but, in some cases, protocol driven administration of thrombolytic therapy is undertaken by nurse practitioners. This has been shown to be both safe and effective at reducing delays. This system is heavily dependent on the training and experience of the staff involved.

Appropriately trained health care professionals should administer thrombolytic therapy with the minimum of delay.

ANGIOPLASTY AND REPERFUSION

9.13 Who should be considered for primary angioplasty?

Primary angioplasty is the first line treatment of choice for all patients presenting with an acute ST-segment elevation myocardial infarction. The widespread use of primary angioplasty is limited by many factors.

Percutaneous coronary intervention for acute myocardial infarction is an expensive treatment that requires the provision of major health care resources and experienced personnel with the necessary expertise. This therapy is, therefore, not available to the majority of patients, particularly those in the district general hospitals where on-site angioplasty is not available.

Currently, many countries do not have the appropriate provision for primary angioplasty. Therefore, many patients receive thrombolysis rather than PCI. This has led several investigators to examine whether patients in centres without the provision for PCI should be treated with thrombolytic therapy alone, transferred immediately to a centre to have PCI, or both (so-called 'facilitated angioplasty').

For some patients, there are contraindications to thrombolytic therapy, such as recent major surgery. Under such circumstances, primary angioplasty should be considered. It should be remembered that PCI requires the administration of potent antiplatelet agents and anticoagulants that may also cause significant bleeding risks.

9.14 What is the evidence for primary angioplasty?

A meta-analysis of 23 randomised trials ($n = 7739$) has demonstrated the superiority of PCI in comparison to streptokinase and fibrin-specific thrombolysis. In comparison to thrombolytic therapy, emergency PCI reduced death (5% versus 7%), non-fatal re-infarction (3% versus 7%), stroke (1% versus 2%), and the combination (8% versus 14%).[7]

There is some evidence to suggest that patients with acute myocardial infarction would benefit from transfer to a centre for primary angioplasty when transfer times are <90 minutes. This benefit is predominantly driven by the subsequent reduction in re-infarction rates rather than mortality.

Some small scale trials have been conducted to look at 'facilitated angioplasty' where thrombolysis is given and the patient immediately transferred for PCI. This may be a promising approach but requires further formal assessment in large scale randomised trials.

9.15 How is reperfusion assessed?

Reperfusion can be assessed in several ways. The simplest method of assessing the response to therapy is the beneficial clinical effects on the patient's progress such as the relief of chest pain and improvements in bradycardia or hypotension. Although the clinical response is important, it cannot be relied upon to provide an accurate assessment of reperfusion. However, the electrocardiogram can provide a sensitive and specific non-invasive method of assessing reperfusion. This is routinely performed at 90–120 minutes after the initiation of thrombolytic therapy.

The restoration of coronary artery patency is usually associated with a >50% reduction in ST-segment elevation or resolution of acute bundle branch block. On occasions, reperfusion is associated with a transient increase in pain and ST-segment elevation before rapid resolution of the ST-segments and relief of symptoms. This is thought to reflect reperfusion injury and is likely to result from a combination of distal embolisation of proximal thrombus and the release of potent vasoactive mediators.

The >50% resolution of ST-segment elevation is approximately 70% specific and 90% sensitive for reperfusion. The specificity for reperfusion increases to nearly 100% with the onset of an accelerated idioventricular rhythm. However, this is not a common occurrence and, therefore, has very poor sensitivity.

The gold standard of assessing reperfusion is coronary angiography. However, outside of the clinical research setting, this is only performed when PCI is being contemplated as a primary or rescue procedure.

Retrospective determination of reperfusion can be established by documenting the release profile of cardiac enzymes and markers. The size of the myocardial infarction is proportional to the area under the curve for serum creatine kinase concentration over the first 48–72 hours. The release of creatine kinase from the infarcted myocardium is damped as an obvious consequence of coronary artery occlusion. With reperfusion, the creatine kinase is 'washed out' of the infarcted territory. This generates a very different creatine kinase temporal profile, such that the peak creatine kinase concentration is much higher but the area under the curve smaller than a similar sized infarct without reperfusion. Modelling of the release kinetics can be used to assess coronary reperfusion.

9.16 What should be done for patients who fail to reperfuse with thrombolytic therapy?

The non-invasive assessment of reperfusion with the 12 lead electrocardiogram is a very useful tool in the assessment of coronary reperfusion following administration of thrombolysis. However, the question of what action should be taken in patients who fail to reperfuse currently has no definitive answer. Three main approaches can be considered: conservative treatment with maintenance antiplatelet and anticoagulant therapy, readministration of thrombolytic therapy or 'rescue' angioplasty.

When there is no evidence of reperfusion after streptokinase administration, some clinicians advocate checking the plasma fibrinogen concentration. If it has not fallen below 1 g/L then this is taken as evidence of failed fibrin(ogen)olysis and tissue plasminogen activator is administered as 'rescue' therapy. Whilst a logical approach, the clinical evidence base is very small and the true clinical benefit unknown, especially given the significant time delays of such an approach.

Percutaneous coronary intervention is sometimes considered in patients who fail to reperfuse with thrombolytic therapy: so-called 'rescue' angioplasty. Rescue angioplasty is predominantly considered in patients who have demonstrated a failure to reperfuse with thrombolytic therapy within 6 hours of symptom onset. The recent REACT trial has suggested that repeat thrombolysis is harmful but 'rescue angioplasty' improves outcome.

SECONDARY PREVENTION IN MYOCARDIAL INFARCTION

9.17 Should β-blockers and ACE inhibitors be administered early in patients with acute myocardial infarction?

Both β-blockers and ACE inhibitors have proven long term secondary preventative benefits in patients who have sustained an acute myocardial infarction. However, the timing of the introduction of these therapies in the peri-infarct period needs to be considered.

β-BLOCKERS

In the first ISIS trial ($n = 16\ 027$),[8] early (mean of 5 hours from symptom onset) intravenous atenolol was associated with a modest relative risk reduction of 15% in 7-day vascular mortality. Post hoc analysis suggests that this mortality benefit is due to a reduction in the risk of cardiac rupture and tamponade (*see Q. 9.22*). Early β-blockade also appears to reduce the combined endpoint of death, cardiac arrest or re-infarction.

The ISIS-1 trial was performed before the introduction of thrombolysis. Some clinicians have questioned whether the modest reductions in the events seen with early intravenous β-blockade are applicable to patients who receive the substantial benefits of thrombolytic therapy. The TIMI-IIB ($n = 1434$)[9] study attempted to address this issue. Patients with acute myocardial infarction were given thrombolysis with tissue plasminogen activator and randomised to early intravenous (within 2 hours of thrombolysis) or delayed oral (day 6) metoprolol. The 7-day mortality was similar in both groups although there was a lower incidence of re-infarction and recurrent chest pain in the early β-blocker group. This trial was clearly not adequately powered to address the potential reduction in mortality with early β-blocker therapy. It did, however, confirm morbidity benefits. Subsequent observational studies have also suggested that early β-blocker use is associated with a reduced rate of cerebral haemorrhage (relative risk reduction 31%) in patients treated with tissue plasminogen activator.

In the absence of contraindications such as asthma or heart block, all patients with acute myocardial infarction should be considered for early intravenous β-blockade.

ANGIOTENSIN CONVERTING ENZYME INHIBITION

A meta-analysis ($n = 98\ 496$) of the randomised controlled trials of ACE inhibition[10] following acute myocardial infarction has assessed the time course of the mortality benefits. Initiation of early (within the first 36 hours) ACE inhibition caused a modest reduction in 30-day mortality (relative risk reduction 7%; 95% confidence intervals, 2–11%). There was also a reduction in early heart failure although the incidence of hypotension and renal dysfunction was increased by ACE inhibitor therapy.

In the absence of significant hypotension, ACE inhibitor therapy should be initiated in the first 36 hours of admission with acute myocardial infarction.

COMPLICATIONS OF MYOCARDIAL INFARCTION

9.18 How does acute cardiac failure manifest?

Cardiac failure can result from ventricular dysfunction due to myocardial necrosis (irreversible), myocardial stunning (potentially reversible with slow recovery) and ongoing ischaemia (reversible with rapid recovery). Depending upon the territory of the myocardial ischaemia, the cardiac failure may predominantly affect the right (inferoposterior ischaemia) or left (anterior ischaemia) ventricle. Ischaemic cardiac failure without previous or current infarction is most likely to occur in patients with critical triple-vessel or left main stem coronary artery disease. In such circumstances, a vicious spiral of progressive ischaemia may occur because the reduction in cardiac output and central aortic pressure leads to further coronary hypoperfusion and myocardial ischaemia, resulting in further deterioration of cardiac function. Cardiogenic shock may rapidly ensue.

Acute cardiac failure is usually manifest by impaired myocardial contractility, high filling pressures and pulmonary oedema. However, it should be recognised that pulmonary oedema may not be a prominent feature in some forms of acute cardiac failure following myocardial ischaemia. This is particularly the case with the syndrome of right ventricular infarction in which there is systemic hypotension and elevation of the jugular venous pressure. There is no pulmonary oedema and left atrial pressure is low because of failure of the right ventricle to deliver blood through the pulmonary circulation. In such circumstances, nitrates and diuretics should be avoided and vigorous intravenous fluids employed in an attempt to increase right-sided cardiac output and thus left atrial and systemic arterial pressure. A pulmonary artery catheter may help guide therapy in these circumstances.

9.19 What is cardiogenic shock?

Cardiogenic shock occurs when there is systemic hypoperfusion due to a low cardiac output and relative arterial hypotension. Tachycardia, cold clammy peripheries and oliguria herald its onset. The systolic blood pressure is usually below 90 mmHg but the absolute systemic pressure may vary. For example, a patient with sustained chronic hypertension may have cardiogenic shock with a systolic blood pressure of 110 mmHg.

Cardiogenic shock is an ominous sign in the context of acute myocardial infarction and is associated with 90% in-hospital mortality. The principles of its management are optimisation of the left ventricular filling pressure and reduction of systemic afterload. Short term inotropic agents can be of benefit but increase cardiac work in an already ischaemic and poorly functioning myocardium. Intra-aortic balloon counterpulsation is very helpful and has two main beneficial haemodynamic effects in this setting: the augmentation of diastolic aortic and coronary perfusion pressure, and the reduction in cardiac afterload and myocardial oxygen demand. The insertion of an intra-aortic balloon pump is usually reserved for those patients with major haemodynamic instability, severe ischaemic left ventricular dysfunction or severe refractory angina, especially as a bridge to coronary angiography and definitive coronary revascularisation.

9.20 How should post infarct or refractory unstable angina be treated?

Recurrent ischaemic cardiac chest pain at rest can occur following myocardial infarction and indicates threatened re-occlusion of the infarct-related artery. Patients with post infarct pain or refractory unstable angina should be maintained on medical therapy for unstable angina, considered for glycoprotein IIb/IIIa receptor antagonism and undergo urgent cardiac catheterisation with a view to coronary revascularisation. Patients with exertional angina following an acute coronary syndrome may be considered for in-patient coronary angiography if it is felt that this is warranted.

9.21 How should arrhythmias be treated?

TACHYCARDIAS

Ventricular fibrillation and ventricular tachycardia are common in the context of infarction and ischaemia. Anti-arrhythmic therapy (intravenous amiodarone) is indicated for resistant, persistent or recurrent cases of haemodynamically compromising ventricular arrhythmias. Non-sustained ventricular tachycardia of brief duration and without haemodynamic compromise does not require specific treatment other than the anti-ischaemic therapies already instituted. Accelerated idioventricular rhythm is an encouraging sign as it represents a very specific marker of reperfusion. Sustained ventricular tachycardia, or ventricular tachycardia associated with compromise, merits prompt treatment with DC cardioversion and amiodarone.

The risk of repeated arrhythmia outwith the context of an acute coronary syndrome is very low. A patient with a successfully treated episode of ventricular fibrillation within the first 24 hours of their myocardial infarction has the same prognosis as a patient with a similar sized infarct who did not have ventricular fibrillation. However, if the patient has ongoing critical ischaemia at rest or with exertion that is associated with ventricular tachyarrhythmia, then there is a high risk of life threatening arrhythmia and the patient should be urgently evaluated for possible coronary revascularisation. Moreover, the occurrence of such malignant arrhythmias beyond 48 hours of the acute coronary event is a poor prognostic sign and merits further detailed evaluation and treatment.

Supraventricular tachyarrhythmias may also occur and usually take the form of a sinus tachycardia, atrial flutter or atrial fibrillation. They often occur as a consequence, or precipitant, of acute cardiac failure. They may be treated with β-blockade, digoxin or amiodarone.

BRADYCARDIAS

Bradycardias are most common with ischaemia or infarction affecting the inferior territory. This occurs because the right coronary artery supplies the sinus and atrioventricular nodes and ischaemia causes their dysfunction, leading to sinus bradycardia and all degrees of atrioventricular block. In the absence of haemodynamic compromise, these arrhythmias should be treated conservatively since they are usually transient and respond to anti-ischaemic and reperfusion therapy. When intervention is required then intravenous atropine, isoprenaline or temporary transvenous pacing may be required. In contrast, atrioventricular block complicating anterior myocardial infarction suggests the need for temporary pacing as it reflects major damage to the His–Purkinje system and can lead to asystole.

9.22 What constitutes myocardial rupture?

Following infarction, the myocardium becomes necrotic and may lead to perforation of the wall of the ventricle. This typically occurs between days 2 and 5 after a transmural myocardial infarction, and presents as one of three forms depending on the area of myocardium that has undergone rupture.

CARDIAC TAMPONADE

Acute free wall rupture usually results in catastrophic cardiac tamponade, pulseless electrical activity and death. There have been occasional reports of successful temporary drainage as a bridge to definitive surgical correction but this is exceptionally rare. Equally uncommon is the self-containment of the rupture and the development of a ventricular pseudoaneurysm.

VENTRICULAR SEPTAL DEFECT

Acute intraventricular septal rupture produces an acquired ventricular septal defect. The presence of a new harsh systolic murmur usually alerts the clinician to the underlying cause of the sudden deterioration in the patient's clinical state. It produces acute cardiac failure, pulmonary oedema and a very high jugular venous pressure. The associated mortality is very high (approaching 100%) and, in addition to the treatment for acute cardiac failure and cardiogenic shock, patients should be considered for urgent surgical correction.

PAPILLARY MUSCLE RUPTURE AND ACUTE MITRAL REGURGITATION

Rupture of one of the left ventricular papillary muscles results in acute mitral regurgitation and severe pulmonary oedema, but is less common than septal rupture. It should also be suspected if there is an acute deterioration in combination with a new systolic murmur, although the murmur may be quiet or inaudible, particularly if the regurgitation is torrential. Again, the patient should be treated for cardiac failure and shock with a view to surgical correction.

Acute ischaemic papillary muscle dysfunction can occasionally occur in the absence of myocardial infarction and rupture. Under these circumstances, the mitral regurgitation is not a constant feature and only appears during acute ischaemic episodes.

9.23 How should pericarditis be treated?

Sharp pleuritic chest pain is common after transmural infarction and may be accompanied by a pericardial rub. Anticoagulants (risk of haemopericardium) and non-steroidal anti-inflammatory drugs (increased risk of myocardial rupture) should be avoided. Simple or opiate-based analgesics are appropriate to relieve the discomfort.

 PATIENT QUESTIONS

9.24 How is a heart attack treated?

Heart attacks need to be treated promptly as this can save lives and help recovery. Anyone with a suspected heart attack must call an emergency ambulance and be immediately taken to a hospital for assessment. This usually involves seeing a doctor, having some blood tests taken and having a 'tracing' of the heart recorded (an electrocardiogram, ECG).

Patients who suffer a heart attack are usually given several forms of treatment over the first few days. Immediate treatment consists of giving powerful painkillers, oxygen via a mask, an aspirin to swallow, and 'clot-buster' treatment through a drip (*see Q. 9.25*). Recently, some patients have been receiving a 'balloon stretch' treatment where the blockage in the heart artery is cleared by a balloon. This is called angioplasty but is not available everywhere.

For the first day or two, patients are observed in a coronary care unit while attached to a heart monitor. Sometimes the heart goes into spasm and requires prompt treatment with an electric shock (defibrillation).

After the first day, several medications are started. These drugs have two roles: to help the heart recover and to prevent recurrent heart attacks. Some of these drugs will be given for a couple of days and most will be given as a tablet. When leaving the hospital, patients are usually given an aspirin to thin the blood, a 'statin' to lower the fats in the blood, a 'beta-blocker' to slow and calm the heart, and an 'ACE inhibitor' to help the healing of the heart scar.

Some patients may need to have an angiogram which shows where the heart arteries are narrowed or blocked. Some patients will require angioplasty (*see above*) or open heart surgery (bypass surgery) to restore the blood flow to the heart.

9.25 What are clot-busters?

When the furred up narrowings (atheroma) of the heart (coronary) arteries become inflamed or damaged, a crack can appear and a clot forms. This clot is supposed to help heal the split in the blood vessel wall. However, sometimes this clot continues to grow and blocks off the artery completely. When this happens, the patient has a myocardial infarction (MI) or 'heart attack'.

One very effective treatment is to give 'clot-busters'. These drugs stimulate the blood to produce substances that dissolve the blood clot. In this way, the supply of blood can be restored to the heart and can limit the amount of damage done to the heart muscle. This treatment improves the chances of surviving a heart attack, particularly when given early after the onset of symptoms (within 6–12 hours). Indeed, the sooner the treatment is given, the better the outcome of the heart attack. This again underlines the importance of seeking medical attention quickly when a heart attack is suspected.

There are potential risks of giving clot-busters. In particular, it increases the risk of internal bleeding including a 1 in 1000 risk of a bleed into the brain. However, overall the considerable benefits outweigh the risks.

The simple drug aspirin also produces similar improvements in patients with a heart attack and should be given to all those with a suspected heart attack. It does not directly dissolve clots, but prevents the clot reforming or getting worse.

9.26 What can or can't I do following a heart attack?

There are no hard and fast rules. However, it is a good time to review how you are looking after yourself and what you can do to lead a healthier life-style (*see below*). Many hospital- and community-based programmes provide clear guidance on what you can do and what to expect after a heart attack.

Exercise does not harm the heart. After a heart attack, it is sensible to increase physical activity slowly and regularly. After the first week of rest, try exercising for 5 minutes a day, usually by taking a walk. This should be increased gradually until you are back to normal activity.

Stress does not cause a heart attack but managing how you deal with stress can help you recover from it. Ensure that after a heart attack you get plenty of rest and relaxation.

Once over the initial convalescent period, many patients return to a full and active life. Many patients actually feel fitter than they were before a heart attack. There is no fixed time for return to engaging in sexual activity. However, once you are able to exercise without limitation, such as climb two flights of stairs, then it is appropriate to start having intercourse again.

It is usually recommended that you should not drive for 1 month after a heart attack. If you are planning air travel then consult your doctor and the airline. Some airline companies refuse to carry patients within 1–3 months of a heart attack.

9.27 How long should I be off work after a heart attack?

Most people are encouraged to stay off work for 4–6 weeks after a heart attack. This period of time can vary depending upon your job and how well you recover. For example, patients with jobs that involve heavy physical activity may need longer to recover than an office worker. Some jobs have strict restrictions. Lorry and bus drivers have to pass further tests before they can return to work (*see Q. 4.16*).

Most patients are seen at a review clinic appointment approximately 4–6 weeks after leaving hospital. The doctor in the clinic will assess your recovery and may perform some tests including putting you on an exercise treadmill (*see Q. 4.15*). At the end of the consultation, the doctor should be in a position to tell you if you can return to work.

When returning to work, it is often best to go back slowly, perhaps working part-time for a while before resuming full work. Discuss this with your doctor and employer.

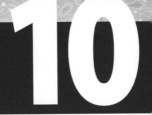

Secondary prevention in patients with CHD

ANTITHROMBOTICS

10.1 What is the indication for aspirin use?

> Aspirin is indicated for the secondary prevention of all forms of coronary heart disease (CHD). Patients with chronic stable angina, unstable angina and myocardial infarction all benefit from aspirin. These benefits are particularly seen with coronary revascularisation: percutaneous coronary intervention (PCI) and coronary artery bypass graft (CABG) surgery. Moreover, aspirin prevents cardiovascular events in patients with cerebrovascular and peripheral vascular disease.

10.2 What are the contraindications to aspirin use?

Aspirin therapy is contraindicated in patients with an aspirin allergy. A proper history should be obtained as allergic reactions are often over-reported and may not represent a true allergy. This is particularly important where a potentially life saving treatment, such as aspirin, is involved. In patients with a clear history of facial swelling and laryngeal oedema, aspirin should not be administered. In the absence of severe symptoms, and where doubt exists, re-challenging the patient may be appropriate.

There are several relative contraindications that reflect the adverse effects of aspirin. The decision to use aspirin depends upon the relative risks and benefits of therapy. The major hazards of aspirin treatment relate to an increased risk of bleeding complications or gastric ulceration. Patients at increased risk of bleeding include those with peptic ulcer disease, history of gastrointestinal haemorrhage, intracranial haemorrhage, concomitant oral anticoagulants and uncontrolled hypertension. Care should be taken when administering aspirin to people taking other non-steroidal anti-inflammatory drugs because this increases the risk of gastrointestinal problems and may lessen the benefit of aspirin.

In patients undergoing surgery, aspirin should be continued in the perioperative period as this will reduce perioperative cardiovascular complications and events. However, if the risks of bleeding are unacceptably high, aspirin should be withdrawn 5–7 days before surgery.

In occasional patients, aspirin can exacerbate asthma. Again, the risks and benefits should be considered but the vast majority of patients with asthma are able to tolerate aspirin well and should not be denied the preventative benefits of aspirin in the presence of concomitant vascular disease.

Where aspirin is contraindicated, clopidogrel is an appropriate alternative (see below).

10.3 What are its adverse effects?

As with all effective antiplatelet agents, there is a small but significant increased risk of bleeding associated with aspirin use. For secondary prevention in patients with CHD, these risks are invariably outweighed by the major benefits of avoiding cardiovascular events (*see Q. 6.33*).

There are theoretical risks of aspirin therapy in patients with asthma and bronchospasm. In a minority of patients, this can create major problems in the control of their respiratory disease. This can occur in patients with severe acute and recurrent exacerbations, mediated through the unwanted effects of aspirin on leukotrienes. Inhibition of potential bronchial relaxation can have adverse effects. However, the majority of patients with asthma, irrespective of disease severity, tolerate aspirin well without deterioration in bronchial reactivity.

10.4 What is the evidence base for its use?

There have been many randomised controlled trials of aspirin use in cardiovascular disease. This evidence base is substantial and the benefits incontrovertible in the context of CHD.

The Antiplatelet Trialists' Collaboration[1] performed the definitive meta-analysis of aspirin use, reporting a relative reduction in the future risk of cardiovascular events and a reduction in the incidence of non-fatal myocardial infarction (*see Q. 6.34*). These benefits were consistently seen across the broad spectrum of CHD, including patients with chronic stable angina, unstable angina and myocardial infarction, and aspirin therapy has been shown to have particular benefits in patients who have undergone coronary revascularisation – either PCI or CABG surgery.

10.5 What alternative antiplatelet agents are there?

Aspirin is a relatively weak antiplatelet agent and this has encouraged the development of more effective antiplatelet agents (*Fig. 10.1*).[2] There are three main classes of antiplatelet agent in addition to aspirin: dipyridamole, thienopyridines and glycoprotein IIb/IIIa receptor antagonists (*see Q. 6.35*). The latter two are discussed below (*see Qs 10.6 and 10.7*).

Dipyridamole is both a vasodilator and antiplatelet agent. It acts through inhibition of platelet phosphodiesterase and thereby blocks cyclic adenosine monophosphate conversion to adenosine triphosphate. This leads to inhibition of platelet adhesion, aggregation and lengthening of shortened platelet survival time. It does not appear to prevent cardiovascular events in patients with CHD. There is some limited evidence from a single large trial, the European Stroke Prevention Study 2, that combination dipyridamole and aspirin therapy may have a role in cerebrovascular disease. In meta-analyses, dipyridamole plus aspirin reduced vascular events but not deaths,

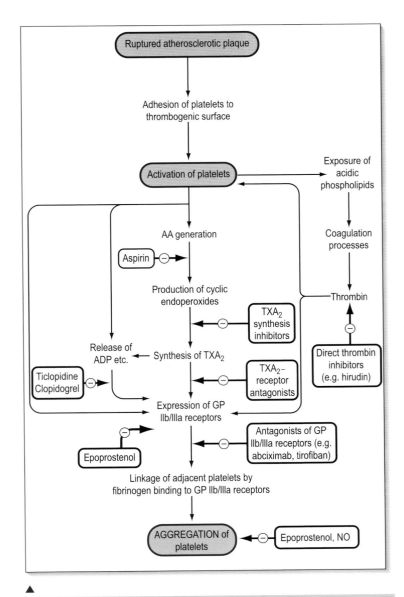

Fig. 10.1 Mechanism of action of various antiplatelet agents. AA, arachidonic acid; ADP, adenosine diphosphate; GP, glycoprotein; NO, nitric oxide; TXA$_2$, thromboxane A$_2$ (Adapted from Rang et al.[2] with permission of Elsevier.)

largely due to the influence of the European Stroke Prevention Study 2 results.

The Antiplatelet Trialists' Collaboration has clearly established that dipyridamole does not have any role in the primary or secondary prevention or treatment of CHD.

10.6 How do thienopyridines work and when should they be used?

There are two main agents in this class: ticlopidine and clopidogrel (*see Q. 6.35*). Ticlopidine is no longer widely used in clinical practice for long term therapy because it has a small (1–2%) but significant risk of inducing potentially fatal neutropenia and agranulocytosis. This bone marrow toxicity is not a feature of clopidogrel, an analogue of ticlopidine.

The current evidence concerning the use of clopidogrel is summarised in *Question 6.36* and indications for its use are given in *Box 10.1*. Current guidelines recommend the use of combined clopidogrel and aspirin therapy in patients with unstable angina or non-ST segment elevation myocardial infarction for at least 9 months. The majority of the benefits are, however, seen in the first 3 months. For patients who have undergone intracoronary stent implantation, previous practice was to administer combination clopidogrel and aspirin therapy for 4 weeks. However, recent evidence from the CREDO trial ($n = 2116$) suggests that this may be too short and many clinicians are now recommending longer treatment (2–12 months) after coronary intervention, especially where drug eluting stents have been employed.

10.7 Is there a role for long term glycoprotein IIb/IIIa receptor antagonists?

The glycoprotein IIb/IIIa receptor is the final common pathway through which platelets aggregate (*see Fig. 10.1*). Whilst these agents will prevent platelet aggregation whatever the stimulus, they do not inhibit platelet activation and degranulation.

The different types of glycoprotein IIb/IIIa receptor antagonist are described in *Question 6.35*.

BOX 10.1 Indications for the use of clopidogrel

■ Secondary prevention of coronary heart disease in patients where aspirin is contraindicated, poorly tolerated or associated with unacceptable side-effects

■ Combination therapy with aspirin in patients with unstable angina or non-ST segment elevation myocardial infarction

■ Combination therapy with aspirin in patients who have undergone PCI and stent implantation

Glycoprotein IIb/IIIa receptor antagonists do not appear to have a role in the long term prevention or treatment of patients with CHD. In the SYMPHONY trial (n = 9233),[3] sibrafiban (low and high dose) was compared to aspirin in patients with a recent acute coronary syndrome. There was no difference in cardiovascular event rates between the three groups although sibrafiban was associated with an ~1.5-fold increased risk of major bleeding.

In the second SYMPHONY trial (n = 6671),[4] patients with a recent acute coronary syndrome were randomised to aspirin alone, high dose sibrafiban alone or aspirin plus low dose sibrafiban for at least 12 months. The trial was terminated early because of the results of the first SYMPHONY trial. There was no difference in the primary endpoint of the trial for the three treatment groups. However, sibrafiban was again associated with an increased bleeding risk but only when used in combination with aspirin. Of major concern, high dose sibrafiban increased both mortality (odds ratio (OR) 1.83; 95% confidence intervals (CI), 1.17–2.88) and the rate of myocardial infarction (OR 1.32; 95% CI, 1.03–1.69) in comparison to aspirin alone. There was also a similar trend with low dose sibrafiban plus aspirin therapy.

In summary, glycoprotein IIb/IIIa receptor antagonists have no role in the secondary prevention of CHD in patients already receiving aspirin or clopidogrel therapy.

10.8 Do oral anticoagulants have benefits?

There have been several studies to assess the efficacy of anticoagulants in the secondary prevention of CHD. These have principally employed warfarin as either a fixed low dose regimen or dose adjusted to maintain therapeutic anticoagulation. A meta-analysis of over 20 000 patients with CHD has shown a clear benefit of oral anticoagulants in the secondary prevention of CHD[5] (*see Box 10.2*).

10.9 Should warfarin be given long term?

As detailed above, there is convincing evidence that oral anticoagulation has significant secondary preventative benefits in patients with CHD even in the absence of atrial fibrillation. The widespread uptake of warfarin has been limited and unpopular because of the implications of therapy and monitoring as well as the major bleeding risk. The use of lower intensity anticoagulation regimens (INR <2.0) combined with aspirin is associated with loss of secondary preventative efficacy whilst maintaining the bleeding risk. Thus where there is concern about the bleeding risks, combination therapy should be avoided and isolated aspirin or clopidogrel considered.

The bleeding risks are largely driven by warfarin rather than aspirin and only patients with a low bleeding risk should be considered for warfarin therapy. Although warfarin plus aspirin is more effective than aspirin alone, it remains unclear whether it is better than warfarin alone. As with atrial

BOX 10.2 Data concerning the benefits of oral anticoagulation

■ *Oral anticoagulation versus control*: In 13 trials (*n* = 8140), high intensity anticoagulation (INR >2.8) was compared to an inactive control.[5] In these studies, oral anticoagulation produced a dramatic reduction in cardiovascular death, myocardial infarction or stroke from 30.3 to 20.3% (RRR 42%; 95% CI, 36–48%). However, this was associated with a marked increase in bleeding risk from 0.7 to 4.6% (odds ratio 4.5; 95% CI, 2.5–6.0). Lower intensities of anticoagulation (INR 2.0–3.0) have not been shown to provide significant preventative benefits but do lead to an increased risk of major bleeding.

■ *Oral anticoagulation versus aspirin*: In six trials (*n* = 4155), oral anticoagulation had significant additional benefits in comparison to aspirin alone. The rate of death, myocardial infarction and stroke was 13.5% on oral anticoagulation and 16.3% on aspirin (RRR 21%; 95% CI, 6–33%). This was associated with a 2.1-fold increased risk of major bleeding.

■ *Oral anticoagulation plus aspirin versus aspirin alone*: The combination of aspirin and oral anticoagulation also has additive benefits as demonstrated in seven trials totalling 12 333 patients. In comparison to aspirin alone, the rate of cardiovascular death, myocardial infarction and stroke was reduced from 17.6 to 15.9% (RRR 12%; 95% CI, 3–20%). Major bleeding events occurred in 3.0% compared with 1.7% respectively, a 1.74-fold increase.

■ *Oral anticoagulation plus aspirin versus oral anticoagulation alone*: As with aspirin alone, oral anticoagulation plus aspirin appears to be better than oral anticoagulation alone. However, the data are limited and involve only three trials incorporating 3142 patients. While the RRR for cardiovascular death, myocardial infarction and stroke appears to be comparable (14%; 95% CI, 6% to +30%) this did not achieve statistical significance (p = 0.15). The major bleeding risks appeared to be very similar: 2.2% for combination therapy compared with 2.3% for oral anticoagulation alone.

■ *Other oral agents*: The recent ESTEEM trial (*n* = 1883) examined the benefits of ximelagatran, a novel oral direct thrombin inhibitor, in patients with a myocardial infarction. Ximelagatran has the advantage that its pharmacodynamic effects are more predictable and, unlike warfarin, it does not require regular monitoring or dose adjustments. This trial also demonstrated a significant reduction from 16.3 to 12.7% (RRR 24%; 95% CI, 2–41%) in the risk of death, recurrent myocardial infarction or severe myocardial ischaemia. Major bleeding events were again increased from 0.9 to 1.8%, a 1.97-fold increase.

CI, confidence intervals; INR, international normalised ratio; RRR, relative risk reduction.

fibrillation, the benefits must be balanced with the major bleeding risks. For many patients, the latter is a major consideration. Warfarin, used alone or in combination with aspirin, may be considered in patients who are at very high cardiovascular risk or who have sustained recurrent cardiovascular events despite aspirin therapy.

Recently, direct oral thrombin inhibitors have been developed that have a more predictable therapeutic range and do not require monitoring of the prothrombin time. Ximelagatran is the first such inhibitor that is now in advanced phase III clinical trials. It is likely that ximelagatran will have very similar secondary preventative benefits in CHD to warfarin but this remains to be established.

STATINS

10.10 How do statins work?

Statins inhibit the enzyme hydroxy-3-methyl glutaryl coenzyme A (HMG CoA) reductase. This is the rate-limiting enzyme in the cholesterol synthetic pathway and converts HMG CoA to mevalonate. Inhibition of the HMG CoA reductase enzyme with statins causes marked reductions in cholesterol synthesis and reduces total and low density lipoprotein (LDL) cholesterol concentrations. Some agents also have modest beneficial effects on increasing high density lipoprotein (HDL) cholesterol concentrations and reducing triglyceride concentrations. The reduction in serum cholesterol concentrations produces marked beneficial clinical effects by reducing plaque progression and atherogenesis.

Recently, there has been interest in the cholesterol-independent effects of statins: their so-called 'pleiotropic effects'. Several lines of evidence suggest that statins may directly affect other pathways involved in atherogenesis: these include improving endothelial function, decreasing vascular inflammation and enhancing plaque stability. There are also intriguing observations suggesting that statins may have very diverse effects such as the prevention of osteoporosis. The role and importance of these pleiotropic effects remain to be established.

10.11 What are the benefits of statins?

Statins potently inhibit the synthesis of cholesterol and reduce serum total and LDL cholesterol concentrations. This inhibits plaque growth and leads to plaque stabilisation. Several observational studies have demonstrated that statins reduce lipid-rich pools and thicken the fibrous cap of atherosclerotic plaques. This leads to plaque stabilisation and a consequent reduction in cardiovascular events, myocardial infarction and death.

Across the spectrum of atherosclerotic disease (coronary heart disease, cerebrovascular disease and peripheral vascular disease), patients benefit from statin therapy. Long term statin therapy is associated with major reductions in the risk of non-fatal myocardial infarction, coronary death, stroke and coronary revascularisation.

10.12 What are the indications for statin therapy?

There have been several large scale, randomised controlled trials to address the issue of lipid lowering therapy in patients with CHD. The 4S trial ($n = 4444$)[6] was the first to demonstrate a significant improvement (relative risk reduction (RRR) 30%) in mortality with the use of simvastatin in patients with CHD and a serum cholesterol concentration greater than 5.5 mmol/L. These mortality benefits have subsequently been shown not only with simvastatin but also with pravastatin. Primary and secondary preventative benefits have also been demonstrated with atorvastatin, fluvastatin and lovastatin.

At present, the goal of therapy would appear to be suppression of the serum total cholesterol concentration to at least below 5.0 mmol/L. The CARE ($n = 4159$), LIPID ($n = 9014$), MIRACL ($n = 3086$) and Heart Protection ($n = 20\ 536$) studies have additionally suggested that patients with average cholesterol concentrations or lower should also be considered for lipid lowering therapy as it is associated with similar relative risk reductions in future adverse cardiac events. However, the target cholesterol seems unclear (*see Q. 10.13*).

10.13 What is the target cholesterol concentration with statin therapy?

At present, there are no clear evidence-based data to address this question. Historically, the randomised controlled trials arbitrarily chose 5.0 mmol/L as the target of total cholesterol concentration. However, the studies do not permit us to determine if 5.5 mmol/L is adequate or if 4.5 and lower will achieve further benefits. At present, the Joint British Cardiac, Diabetic, Hypertension and Hyperlipidaemia Societies currently recommend that all patients with CHD should receive statin therapy with the target of reducing their serum total cholesterol below 5.0 mmol/L. It is likely that this threshold concentration will be reduced further. However, there are strong arguments to lower the cholesterol whatever the absolute serum cholesterol concentration. The data from the CARE, HPS, MIRACL and ASCOT-LLA trials suggest it is the overall absolute risk that is important rather than the cholesterol concentration per se. If a patient is at high risk, they will benefit from cholesterol reduction irrespective of their cholesterol concentration. For example, in the Heart Protection Study,[7] patients with a total cholesterol concentration less than 5.0 mmol/L had a 5-year event rate of

22.1% that was reduced to 16.9% by simvastatin 40 mg daily. Thus a patient with a recent myocardial infarction, diabetes mellitus and peripheral vascular disease will merit statin therapy even if their total cholesterol concentration is 3.6 mmol/L.

Some authorities have argued that the secondary preventative benefits of statins are independent of the serum cholesterol reductions and it is the pleiotropic effects of statins that account for their clinical utility. This, however, seems unlikely. There are several ongoing trials that are assessing whether more intensive lipid lowering with low and high dose or potency statins will lead to improved clinical outcomes. These trials will help us to guide the approach to cholesterol reduction in patients with CHD. A recent meta-analysis incorporating ~28 000 patients has suggested that greater reductions in serum LDL cholesterol concentrations are associated with more marked secondary preventative benefits.

There are some data from a randomised controlled trial that more intensive lipid lowering therapy will have additional benefits. Patients who have undergone saphenous vein bypass grafting appear to gain more benefit from intensive reductions in serum LDL cholesterol concentrations. In the Post Coronary Artery Bypass Graft trial ($n = 1351$), progression of atherosclerosis or vascular occlusion was reduced in patients treated to a serum LDL cholesterol concentration of <2.6 mmol/L compared to those treated to ~3.5 mmol/L. This was translated into reductions of clinical events including recurrent revascularisation.

Recently the PROVE-IT trial ($n = 4162$) demonstrated that more intensive lipid-lowering therapy with atorvastation 80 mg was superior to more modest cholesterol reduction with pravastatin 40 mg daily. This would appear to suggest that intensive cholesterol reduction is more beneficial, especially where LDl cholesterol is ≥3.2 mmol/L.

10.14 What are the contraindications to statin therapy?

Statins are generally very well tolerated with few adverse effects. The main contraindications of statins relate to their potential adverse effects on the liver and skeletal muscle that may be increased by other concomitant medications such as fibrates. Other contraindications include women of child-bearing potential, pregnancy, breast feeding and porphyria.

Statin therapy can lead to elevations in liver enzymes, particularly transaminases. Patients with active liver disease should, therefore, not receive statin therapy. Transient rises in the transaminases are common early after initiation of statin therapy but rarely (<1%) rise above three times the upper limit of normal. It is recommended that liver function tests are documented before initiating treatment and monitored for at least the first few months of therapy.

10.15 What are their adverse effects?

 Statins can occasionally cause myopathy. This may be manifest as generalised myalgia with or without elevation in skeletal muscle enzymes, such as creatine kinase. Many patients complain of tiredness and myalgia on routine inquiry. Statins should not be discontinued unless there is a clear causal association between drug and symptoms. Trial withdrawal of therapy and re-challenging with the statin may be appropriate. In the Heart Protection Study,[7] myalgia was reported by 32.9% of patients allocated simvastatin and 33.2% of patients allocated placebo.

Myositis and rhabdomyolysis are very rare but important adverse effects. Elevation of the creatine kinase 10 times the upper limit of normal occurs in 0.1% of patients and rhabdomyolysis in ~0.05%. In the randomised controlled trials, these rates are very similar to those seen in patients taking placebo (0.06% and 0.03% respectively). Although the adverse effects of statins are rapidly reversible on discontinuation of therapy, statin-induced rhabdomyolysis has ~10% mortality. Patients with a known prior or current myopathy should not receive statin therapy.

10.16 How soon after an acute coronary syndrome should statins be administered?

It should be recognised that patients presenting with an acute coronary syndrome will experience a fall in their serum cholesterol concentrations as a consequence of the acute illness which can last for up to 3 months. It is, therefore, preferable to assess the serum lipid profile within 24 hours of symptom onset. Patients should not have been judged to reach their target cholesterol until after at least 12 weeks of convalescence.

The original statin trials (4S, CARE, LIPID) excluded patients who had an acute coronary syndrome within 4–6 months. This exclusion was imposed because of the uncertain safety profile of this class of drug. Following the publication of the landmark trials, the question of whether it was safe or indeed beneficial to introduce statin therapy early after an acute coronary syndrome was resolved by observational studies which suggested that early statin use was associated with major reductions in subsequent and early recurrent cardiovascular events.

The MIRACL trial ($n = 3086$)[8] recruited patients within 4 days of an acute coronary syndrome and randomised them to atorvastatin 80 mg daily or placebo for 16 weeks. Patients with significant hypercholesterolaemia (>7.0 mmol/L) were excluded but there was no lower limit of cholesterol concentration for inclusion in the trial. Although this was a very short term trial (16 weeks compared to the 5 years of previous trials), there was a significant reduction in the primary endpoint from 17.4 to 14.8% ($p = 0.048$). This benefit was largely driven by a reduction in recurrent severe ischaemia requiring re-hospitalisation (8.4 to 6.2%; RRR 24%, p = 0.02). This result is, in some ways, remarkable given the very brief period of treatment. This indicates that not only is statin therapy safe immediately after an acute coronary syndrome but it is also probably beneficial if given early. This presumably reflects the advantageous remodelling effects of lipid lowering therapy following acute plaque rupture.

Statins should be administered early after a patient presents with an acute coronary syndrome.

10.17 Are there differences between drugs in this class?

There are several important differences between the types of statin therapy.

EFFICACY

The reduction in serum cholesterol concentrations varies markedly between the types of statin. Comparative trials have indicated that significant differences exist (*Table 10.1*). Pravastatin and fluvastatin appear to produce modest reductions in serum cholesterol concentrations, simvastatin and lovastatin cause moderate reductions whereas atorvastatin and rosuvastatin lead to the greatest reductions in cholesterol concentrations.

EVIDENCE BASE

The statins that have been assessed in major randomised controlled trials of primary and secondary prevention are:

- Pravastatin – WOSCOPS, CARE and LIPID trials
- Simvastatin – 4S and HPS trials
- Atorvastatin – ASCOT-LLA and MIRACL trials
- Fluvastatin – LIPS and FLARE trials
- Lovastatin – AFCAPs/TEXCAPs trial.

TABLE 10.1 Reduction in baseline serum LDL cholesterol concentrations

Statin	Daily dose			
	10 mg	20 mg	40 mg	80 mg
Fluvastatin	15%	21%	27%	33%
Pravastatin	20%	24%	29%	33%
Lovastatin	21%	29%	37%	45%
Simvastatin	27%	32%	37%	42%
Atorvastatin	37%	43%	49%	55%
Rosuvastatin	43%	48%	53%	58%*

*Rosuvastatin 80 mg is currently unlicensed because of safety concerns.

SAFETY

The incidence of serious adverse effects is not the same for all statins. This, in part, reflects how the different statins are metabolised.

Simvastatin can interact with drugs that inhibit the cytochrome P_{450} 3A4 enzyme and these include phenazone, propranolol, digoxin and warfarin and other coumarin derivatives. To avoid potential interactions, simvastatin is often given late in the evening. Cerivastatin has a similar and more marked interaction with the cytochrome P_{450} 3A4 enzyme. This interaction led to a much higher incidence of statin-associated rhabdomyolysis and resulted in the recent withdrawal of cerivastatin from the market. Cerivastatin was responsible for more than half of all the reported cases of rhabdomyolysis.

There are now extensive safety data on most statins and there is clear evidence that the current evidence-based statins are safe and have a good side-effect profile.

10.18 When should other (non-statin) lipid lowering agents be considered?

There are many non-statin agents that lower cholesterol concentrations: fibrates, resins, niacin, ezetimibe. However, although these drugs lower serum lipid concentrations, they have not been clearly shown to reduce mortality in randomised controlled trials. These agents are usually reserved for patients who have contraindications to statin therapy or are used as adjunctive therapy in patients who have resistant hypercholesterolaemia despite statin therapy. It should be remembered that the adverse effects of statins are potentiated by other lipid lowering therapies.

■ *Fibrates* have a direct action on the liver to reduce triglyceride concentrations and, to a variable extent, LDL cholesterol concentrations. They may also increase HDL cholesterol concentrations and may be particularly useful in those patients with low HDL cholesterol concentrations. In the VA-HIT trial ($n = 2531$),[9] gemfibrozil 1.2 g daily had modest benefits in patients with CHD and a normal LDL cholesterol concentration (≤ 3.7 mmol/L) but a reduced HDL cholesterol concentration (≤ 1.0 mmol/L). Its use was associated with a 22% relative risk reduction (95% CI, 7–35%) in major adverse cardiac events but no effect on overall mortality.

■ *Resins*, such as colestyramine and colestipol, bind bile acids and prevent their intestinal reabsorption. This promotes bile acid synthesis and reduces LDL cholesterol concentrations. This may be used in association with other therapies to reduce serum cholesterol concentrations but their use is associated with extensive gastrointestinal side-effects and may adversely increase triglyceride concentrations.

■ *Niacin and nicotinic acid derivatives* are limited by the marked side-effects which include vasodilatation, flushing, rashes and gastrointestinal upset. These agents produce very modest effects on lipid levels.

■ *Ezetimibe* is a new class of lipid lowering therapy that acts through reductions in intestinal cholesterol absorption. It is currently indicated as adjunctive therapy in patients with resistant hypercholesterolaemia.

β-BLOCKERS

10.19 What are the benefits of β-blockers?

β-blockers are antagonists at β-adrenoceptors, and thus produce negative chronotropism and negative inotropism in the heart. The attenuation of the heart rate response to exercise and stress reduces the myocardial oxygen demand and severity of ischaemia. It also prolongs diastole, a major determinant of myocardial perfusion time. Randomised controlled trials have demonstrated that β-blocker therapy is efficacious in reducing symptoms of angina, episodes of ischaemia and improving exercise capacity.

The indications for β-blockers are expanding. There is clear evidence that β-blockade has major morbidity and mortality benefits in patients with myocardial infarction and chronic heart failure, reducing the risk of recurrent myocardial infarction and death.

10.20 What are their adverse effects?

 True side-effects from β-blocker therapy are uncommon (<10%) but do include symptoms, such as fatigue and lethargy, which are commonly encountered on routine enquiry. A causative association should, therefore, be established before permanently discontinuing β-blocker therapy. Because of β-adrenergic receptor upregulation in the presence of β-blockade, patients should not be withdrawn from therapy rapidly. This can cause an acute withdrawal syndrome and there is a suggestion that this may even precipitate acute myocardial infarction.

10.21 What is the evidence base for their use?

Meta-analyses ($n = 54\,234$) have demonstrated that β-blockers have a major benefit in reducing the risk of death by 23% in patients after an acute myocardial infarction.[10] These benefits are demonstrable for at least the first 2 years and are probably sustained beyond this. Hypertension and case-control studies have also shown that patients maintained on β-blockers are less likely to have a major adverse cardiac event and have a reduced mortality if they subsequently suffer a myocardial infarction. For these reasons, β-blockers should be considered in patients with CHD and hypertension.

Hypertension and angina trials indicate that β-blockers are better tolerated and have fewer side-effects than other commonly prescribed agents, such as calcium channel antagonists. Concerns that β-blocker therapy is associated with reduced peripheral perfusion in patients with peripheral vascular disease are unfounded. β-blockers may have significant secondary preventative benefits in these patients as suggested by the marked reductions in perioperative mortality and myocardial infarction when undergoing major vascular surgery.

Because of the common risk factor of smoking, many patients with angina have chronic obstructive pulmonary disease and are denied β-blocker therapy due to the concern of provoking bronchospasm. Observational data demonstrate that patients with obstructive pulmonary disease derive similar mortality benefits (RRR 40%) following myocardial infarction with β-blocker therapy. Therefore, such patients should be given a trial β-blockade since the majority tolerate therapy well. If there is genuine concern of clinically significant reversible bronchospasm, formal spirometry in the presence and absence of a β_2 agonist, such as nebulised salbutamol 5 mg, should be performed.

Patients with ischaemic heart disease and coexisting heart failure are particularly at risk and should also be given β-blocker therapy as the agent of choice. There have been several large scale, randomised controlled trials that have demonstrated major mortality and morbidity benefits in patients with mild to severe heart failure maintained on β-blocker therapy. Metoprolol (MERIT-HF trial, $n = 3991$), carvedilol (programme of trials, $n = 1094$) and bisoprolol (CIBIS II, $n = 2647$) have all been shown to reduce mortality by at least 34% in patients with heart failure maintained on ACE inhibitor therapy. Despite theoretical and prejudicial concerns, β-blockers improve both morbidity and mortality in this important group of patients. There is, however, concern with regard to the initiation of therapy in patients with heart failure because of the potential to precipitate acute decompensation. It is currently recommended that β-blockade is initiated slowly with a cautious uptitration over a 6–8 week period. Several initiatives are being explored in order to facilitate this uptitration phase including heart failure liaison nurses and starter packs.

10.22 Are there differences between drugs in this class?

There is no evidence to support the suggestion that one type of β-blocker is superior to another. The so-called highly selective β_1 blockers (e.g. celiprolol or bisoprolol), or those with combined vasodilating and antioxidant properties (e.g. carvedilol), have no proven benefits above conventional β-blockers (e.g. atenolol or metoprolol). However, the secondary preventative benefits of β-blockers may be lost where agents have intrinsic sympathomimetic action and the use of such agents should, therefore, be avoided.

The COMET trial ($n = 3029$)[11] did compare two β-blockers, carvedilol and metoprolol, in the treatment of chronic heart failure. There was a modest favourable effect of carvedilol in comparison to metoprolol. However, this trial used an inappropriately low dose of metoprolol and it cannot be viewed as demonstrating superiority of one β-blocker over another.

10.23 How long should β-blockers be given after myocardial infarction?

This is a contentious area. The trials of β-blockade in patients who had sustained an acute myocardial infarction were conducted before the advent of large scale, randomised controlled trials. Many trials had a limited follow-up and did not assess the long term benefits. The evidence is, therefore, limited to 2 years post myocardial infarction and there is general agreement that β-blockade should be given to all patients for at least the first 2 years after myocardial infarction.

After 2 years, there are differing views as to the merits of continuing β-blockade. Meta-analyses indicate that the benefits are indeed sustained after 2 years and there is no suggestion of loss of benefit over time. Clearly, where there is evidence of significant left ventricular dysfunction, trial evidence would support the use of indefinite β-blocker therapy. However, where there is preserved left ventricular function, continuation of β-blockade beyond 2 years is less clear. It would seem sensible to continue therapy where there is an additional indication, such as hypertension or angina pectoris, or where it is well tolerated. Withdrawal of β-blockade can be associated with major adverse effects.

ACE INHIBITORS

10.24 How do ACE inhibitors work?

Angiotensin converting enzyme (ACE) is present on the endothelial cell surface and converts angiotensin I to angiotensin II. Angiotensin II causes marked arterial vasoconstriction, as well as salt and water retention, leading to an increase in vascular resistance, blood volume and arterial pressure. However, ACE was also identified as an enzyme that metabolises bradykinin. Indeed, it has a higher substrate affinity for bradykinin than angiotensin I. The benefits of ACE inhibition are likely to relate to both the inhibition of the renin–angiotensin–aldosterone system as well as the potentiation of bradykinin action.

Inhibition of ACE has a weak vasodilator and vasodepressor effect. This is particularly marked where there is activation of the renin–angiotensin–

aldosterone system, such as with concomitant potent diuretic therapy. This reduces cardiac afterload and inhibits salt and water retention. There are also potentially beneficial effects on heart rate variability and left ventricular remodelling, particularly after acute myocardial infarction. ACE inhibitors also have beneficial effects on vascular function that improve endothelial dysfunction, enhance endogenous fibrinolysis and reduce vascular inflammation.

10.25 What are the benefits of ACE inhibitors?

All patients with CHD should be considered for maintenance ACE inhibitor therapy because of the major secondary preventative benefits. ACE inhibition is associated with a significant reduction in death, myocardial infarction, stroke, renal failure, diabetes mellitus and hypertension. In particular, ACE inhibition appears to have an anti-ischaemic effect and consistently reduces the risk of myocardial infarction by ~20%.

ACE inhibition produces symptomatic benefits in patients with heart failure and is associated with improvements in New York Heart Association (NYHA) class and exercise capacity. In patients with preserved left ventricular function, ACE inhibition does not have any specific symptomatic benefits but does improve prognosis in patients with a wide range of vascular disease and associated risk factors.

10.26 Should ACE inhibitors only be used in patients with heart failure?

The major morbidity and mortality benefits of ACE inhibitor therapy were first demonstrated in patients who were at the greatest risk – those with overt heart failure. These benefits are, at least in part, likely to reflect an anti-ischaemic action of ACE inhibition, particularly given the reduction in re-infarction rates seen in all the major randomised controlled trials.

The HOPE study ($n = 9297$)[12] was a large scale, randomised controlled trial of ramipril 10 mg daily in patients with vascular disease (55% having chronic stable angina) without heart failure. During the 4.5 years of follow-up, ramipril was associated with reductions in all-cause mortality, myocardial infarction and stroke. Moreover, these beneficial effects appeared to be independent of the associated reductions in blood pressure, and are particularly marked in patients with diabetes mellitus. The EUROPA trial ($n = 12\ 218$)[13] was a large scale, randomised controlled trial of perindopril 8 mg daily in relatively low risk patients with coronary artery disease. After 4 years of follow-up, there was a 20% reduction in the risk of cardiovascular death, myocardial infarction or cardiac arrest.

There is now clear and consistent evidence that ACE inhibition should be given to all patients with coronary artery disease irrespective of left ventricular function. This is associated with a significant reduction in the risk of myocardial infarction: consistent 20–22% relative risk reduction in all trials. The beneficial effects on mortality appear to depend upon the overall cardiovascular risk of the patient: greatest in those with severe left ventricular dysfunction and least in those at low risk with preserved left ventricular dysfunction.

10.27 What are the contraindications to ACE inhibitors?

Angiotensin converting enzyme inhibition should be avoided in patients with critical renovascular disease. Severe renal artery stenosis generates marked elevations in serum renin and angiotensin II concentrations that attempt to sustain renal perfusion pressure. Inhibition of ACE may, therefore, cause marked renal hypoperfusion and renal failure. Unless treatment is protracted or perfusion critical, ACE inhibitor induced renal dysfunction is usually reversible after cessation of therapy.

Occasionally, ACE inhibition may lead to acute precipitous hypotension that can cause dizziness, light-headedness and syncope. This is, however, unusual and can be avoided by longer acting ACE inhibitors, cautious uptitration and nocturnal dosing.

Because of the occasional precipitous hypotension, it is normal practice to avoid ACE inhibitors in patients with severe aortic stenosis. There is no evidence base for this approach and some have argued that ACE inhibition may be of benefit, particularly in those patients with heart failure secondary to severe aortic stenosis. It would seem pertinent to avoid short acting ACE inhibitors that are associated with more marked acute changes in blood pressure, such as captopril. However, cautious introduction of ACE inhibition may have benefits in patients with heart failure due to aortic stenosis. For those patients with critical aortic stenosis unknowingly maintained on long term ACE inhibitor therapy, treatment should be continued unless there are major contraindications or severe side-effects.

ACE inhibition is contraindicated in women of child-bearing potential and in pregnancy. Depending upon the preparation, it should also be avoided in mothers who are breast feeding.

10.28 What are their adverse effects?

 There are several adverse effects of ACE inhibitor therapy. Renal dysfunction is common and, following commencement of therapy, initial monitoring of renal function is mandatory because occasionally renal failure may rapidly ensue. This is usually reversed on discontinuation of therapy.

Hyperkalaemia may occur, especially when co-administered with potassium-sparing diuretics such as spironolactone or triamterene. Rarely, this may lead to serious hyperkalaemia in the presence or absence of renal failure.

Symptomatic hypotension, dizziness and light-headedness are occasional features of ACE inhibition. This usually occurs when initiated in patients with prior relative hypotension or already receiving potent diuretic therapy.

A dry, tickly, non-productive cough is also a characteristic side-effect of ACE inhibition. Its prevalence is probably over-reported. Cough is a common symptom and a clear causative relationship should be established. Many patients with an upper respiratory tract infection have their ACE inhibitor therapy discontinued unnecessarily. However, it can be an intolerable and irritating side-effect for a substantial number of patients; prevalence is 5–10%.

ACE inhibition may be associated with the development of angio-oedema. This is fortunately a very rare occurrence but can be life threatening if orolaryngeal oedema occurs. The incidence of this side-effect appears to be increased in certain ethnic groups (e.g. African-Americans) and the concomitant use of neutral endopeptidase inhibitors.

10.29 What is the evidence base for their use?

There is a large evidence base for ACE inhibition in patients with CHD. The mortality benefits appear to relate to the overall risk of the population. Early trials were performed in high risk patients with heart failure due to left ventricular systolic dysfunction: mortality at 4 years of ~30%. A meta-analysis of the major randomised controlled trials ($n = 12$ 763) demonstrated that ACE inhibition reduced total mortality by 20%.[14] In the HOPE trial ($n = 9297$),[12] patients with moderate risk had a mortality rate of 12% over 4 years and ramipril reduced total mortality by 16%. The recent EUROPA trial ($n = 12$ 218)[13] (*Fig. 10.2*) had a similar risk population with a 4-year mortality rate of 17%. Perindopril reduced total mortality by 14%. However, irrespective of the overall risk, ACE inhibition appears to have a remarkably consistent benefit in reducing the future risk of myocardial infarction: 20–22% relative risk reduction in the rate of myocardial infarction.

Although proportional to overall cardiovascular risk, there is a large evidence base that supports the use of ACE inhibition in all patients with CHD.

10.30 Are there differences between drugs in this class?

There are several important differences between the various ACE inhibitor drugs. The main differences relate to the pharmacokinetics, tissue penetration and evidence base.

PHARMACOKINETICS

Captopril was the first ACE inhibitor to be employed in widespread clinical use. It also has the shortest plasma half-life and is administered two or three

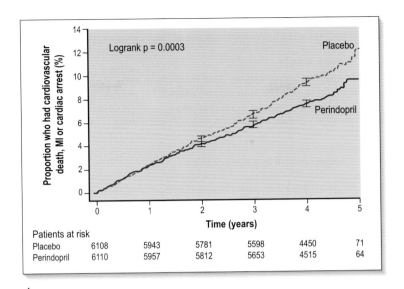

Fig. 10.2 Effects of ACE inhibition in patients with coronary artery disease. Perindopril treatment was associated with a significant reduction in the primary endpoint (cardiovascular mortality, non-fatal myocardial infarction, and resuscitated cardiac arrest; p = 0.0003). (From Fox.[12] Reprinted with permission from Elsevier.)

times daily. This has the potential to have marked peak and trough effects with large swings in blood pressure. Acute captopril dosing is, therefore, more likely to induce symptomatic hypotension and dizziness.

Some agents rely upon a longer acting active metabolite, such as enalapril and enalaprilat, to cause less marked swings in blood pressure. However, newer agents, such as lisinopril, ramipril and perindopril, have a long half-life and produce more gradual but sustained reductions in blood pressure. The latter may be better tolerated and easier to administer in the community.

TISSUE PENETRATION

Some ACE inhibitor agents penetrate tissues less easily. Much has been made about the better and more complete tissue penetration of some ACE inhibitors, such as quinapril, lisinopril and perindopril. Tissue ACE inhibition may be more important for the beneficial effects on factors such as left ventricular hypertrophy and remodelling. Given that ACE is predominantly expressed on the endothelial cell surface, tissue penetration is perhaps overemphasised in terms of the vascular actions of these agents.

EVIDENCE BASE

The early evidence base for ACE inhibitor therapy has predominantly been demonstrated with captopril and enalapril in patients with heart failure. Subsequent trials were performed in patients who had sustained an acute myocardial infarction with or without heart failure. The evidence base was then extended to include lisinopril, ramipril and trandolapril. Recent trials have now included patients without prior infarction or heart failure and included ramipril and perindopril.

10.31 What alternative agents are there?

ACE inhibitor drugs have significant side-effects and are not well tolerated by up to a third of patients. There are alternative therapies that can be used as second line therapy. Angiotensin II type 1 receptor antagonists, so-called angiotensin receptor blockers (ARBs), have been developed as an alternative and potentially more effective approach to inhibiting the renin–angiotensin system.

The early ELITE study ($n = 722$)[15] suggested that the ARB, losartan, had more marked beneficial secondary preventative benefits than the ACE inhibitor, captopril. However, the ELITE II study ($n = 3152$)[16] was unable to confirm these initial tentative findings and losartan was not found to be superior to captopril (*Fig. 10.3*). Indeed, the ELITE II and OPTIMAAL[17] trials suggested a potential superiority of captopril over losartan. In all of these trials, losartan was better tolerated with fewer side-effects than captopril.

The Val-HeFT (valsartan, $n = 5010$) and CHARM-Alternative (candesartan, $n = 2028$) trials have recently assessed the benefits of ARBs in patients with heart failure who are unable to tolerate ACE inhibitor therapy. In these patients, ARBs have significant morbidity and mortality benefits although the magnitude of these benefits appears to be more modest than those associated with ACE inhibitors.

Patients may not be able to tolerate ACE inhibitor therapy not only because of troublesome side-effects but also because of renal dysfunction. While ARBs are appropriate for the former, the ELITE study demonstrated that ARBs cause similar degrees of renal dysfunction as ACE inhibitors. Thus where patients with heart failure are intolerant of ACE inhibitors due to renal dysfunction, ARBs should be avoided and the combination of hydralazine and nitrates considered since this was associated with very modest benefits in the early V-HeFT I ($n = 642$) trial.

There are currently no randomised controlled trials to assess specifically the role of ARBs in patients with CHD and preserved left ventricular dysfunction. The CHARM-Preserved trial ($n = 3023$)[18] randomised patients

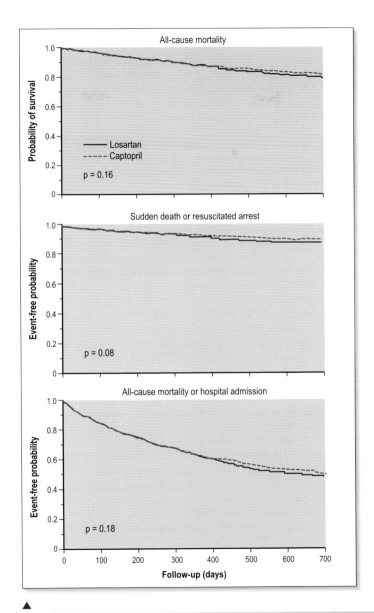

▲

Fig. 10.3 Comparison of losartan and captopril. (From Pitt et al.[16] with permission.)

with symptomatic heart failure and preserved left ventricular function (ejection fraction >40%) to candesartan or placebo. Over half of the patients had CHD as the underlying aetiology of heart failure. Overall, mortality was identical in both groups although candesartan did reduce the frequency of recurrent hospitalisations for heart failure by 18%.

Angiotensin receptor blockers are currently only indicated in patients with CHD if they also have heart failure.

MISCELLANEOUS

10.32 Should hormone replacement therapy be given to postmenopausal women?

Large observational studies have suggested that hormone replacement therapy (HRT), and in particular oestrogen, has a cardioprotective effect in women. However, there are many confounding factors in these observational studies such as the influence of socioeconomic class and motivation in women taking HRT. Moreover, pooled data from ongoing trials have so far failed to demonstrate a significant cardioprotective effect of HRT. The first randomised controlled trial of HRT, the HERS trial ($n = 2763$),[19] failed to demonstrate a benefit with 5 years of HRT in postmenopausal women with CHD. Protagonists have suggested that the HERS trial may indicate an initial adverse effect of HRT which could be offset by protection against future cardiac events with long term (>3 years) sustained therapy. However, the HART trial ($n = 226$) failed to demonstrate a significant effect of HRT on the progression of atherosclerosis on coronary angiography over a 3.3 year follow-up.[20] Finally, the Women's Health Initiative trial ($n = 16\ 608$) failed to demonstrate any benefit of combined HRT in the primary prevention of CHD over 5.2 years of follow-up.[21] Indeed, there was again a suggestion of an increased risk in the first year after commencing HRT.

Hormone replacement therapy has no role in the primary or secondary prevention of CHD and its routine use cannot be advocated. In patients who develop CHD while taking HRT, there is no evidence to suggest a benefit of discontinuing therapy. In women wishing to take HRT because, for example, they may have troublesome symptoms of the menopause, HRT should be administered following clinical assessment and treatment of risk factors for CHD.

10.33 Should antioxidant vitamins be routinely given?

There has been a major interest in the role of oxidation in the pathogenesis of atherosclerosis: specifically, the role of oxidised LDLs in the formation of foam cells and atherosclerotic plaques. Moreover, there has been a large body of promising preclinical data to suggest that supplementation of the diet with antioxidants can markedly inhibit atherogenesis.

Clinical observational cohort studies have also indicated major reductions in mortality and cardiovascular events in people taking antioxidant vitamins. These findings have formed the rationale for major randomised controlled trials of antioxidant vitamins in the primary and secondary prevention of CHD. With the exception of the CHAOS trial,[22] these trials have failed to demonstrate a significant benefit of antioxidant vitamins. The aptly named CHAOS trial changed the dose of vitamin E during the conduct of the trial and the benefits were inconsistent, appearing to reduce only the incidence of non-fatal myocardial infarction.

A recent meta-analysis assessed the effects of vitamin E and β-carotene on long term cardiovascular morbidity and mortality.[23] Data from seven trials of vitamin E incorporating 81 788 patients clearly demonstrated no effect of vitamin E supplementation on the separate endpoints of all-cause mortality, cardiovascular death, stroke or non-fatal myocardial infarction. These findings are consistent for both primary and secondary prevention of CHD.

There were eight major trials that assessed the effects of β-carotene and provided a total sample population of 138 113 patients. Meta-analysis identified no benefit of β-carotene therapy and, of concern, there was a small increased risk of all-cause (OR 1.07; 95% CI, 1.02–1.11) and cardiovascular (OR 1.1; 95% CI, 1.03–1.17) mortality.

Across a broad dose range, there is no consistent evidence to indicate a role of antioxidant vitamins in the secondary prevention of CHD. Indeed, in the case of β-carotene, there may be a small but significant adverse effect.

10.34 What is the evidence for fish oils?

There is increasing evidence to support the role of polyunsaturated fatty (omega-3) acids (docosahexaenoic acid, DHA, and eicosapentaenoic acid, EPA) or fish oils in both the primary and secondary prevention of ischaemic heart disease.

Following the observation that Greenland Eskimos and Japanese fishermen have a low death rate from cardiovascular disease, it was suggested that this could be related to their high dietary intake of fish. In the Seven Countries Study, vegetable foods, alcohol and fish consumption were inversely correlated with CHD mortality. Subsequent observational studies such as the Chicago Western Electric Study, the Zutphen Study and the usual care group in the Multiple Risk Factor Intervention Trial reported an inverse relationship between the daily dietary consumption of oily fish and the death rate from CHD in men. More recently an inverse relationship between fish consumption and omega-3 fatty acid intake and the risk of CHD, and in particular the risk of fatal CHD events, has been reported in women. Not all studies have demonstrated this inverse relationship although some benefit was observed on cardiovascular outcomes, even in individuals with a low habitual intake of oily fish, and this benefit appears to be independent of other risk factors.

In the Physicians' Health Study, the consumption of one or more portions of fish at least once a week was associated with a 52% reduction in the risk of sudden cardiac death, but no relationship was seen between fish consumption and the risk of a first myocardial infarction. This beneficial effect seems to be specific to oily fish since in the Seven Countries Study oily fish consumption of around 15 g/day was associated with a 34% reduction in the risk of ischaemic heart disease death, but there was no association with total or lean fish consumption. In the Honolulu Heart Study, oily fish appeared to offer particular protection to smokers from CHD.

Oily fish have been shown to reduce deaths from ischaemic heart disease in patients following acute myocardial infarction. In the diet and re-infarction (DART) study, the advice to eat at least two portions of oily fish each week was associated with a significant reduction in mortality.[24] Furthermore, the GISSI-Prevenzione investigators demonstrated that a daily capsule containing 1 g of DHA/EPA reduced all-cause mortality and improved cardiovascular outcomes at 42 months.[25] The dose of DHA/EPA was equivalent to fish five times a week. However, it should be recognised that this was not a proper double-blind, randomised controlled trial as there was no placebo therapy and this may have influenced the results.

10.35 What is the role of cardiac rehabilitation?

While cardiac rehabilitation began as an exercise based activity designed to combat the loss of cardiovascular fitness associated with prolonged bed-rest after myocardial infarction, the modern approach to rehabilitation recognises that in addition to the physical element there are psychological and social aspects to the rehabilitation process.

Modern cardiac rehabilitation should be about involving the patient in a process of 'self-management' of a chronic disease process in the same way as one would a diabetic. The aims of that process of rehabilitation are two-fold: first, to modify the disease process (secondary prevention), and second, to assist the patient to return to a 'normal' role in society. It is, therefore, a process of behavioural modification that should encourage adaptive behaviours in the patient which will assist those aims.

Central to the process of rehabilitation are pathology, impairment, disability and handicap (*Box 10.3*).

Much of our management in cardiology is targeted at the levels of pathology and impairment. We prescribe drugs or undertake interventions to modify impairment that we believe to be responsible for the patient's disabilities. We judge our success mainly by the modification of pathology or alleviation of impairment. Given the causal relationship between pathology or impairment, and disability or handicap, we expect that the latter will improve. However, this correlation is relatively low: for example, the patient with minimal coronary disease who complains of intractable angina preventing even light exercise or the patient with an ejection fraction of 15% who denies breathlessness on exertion. Some of the variance may be explained by factors within the organ or the individual (e.g. collateralisation, vasospasm or tolerance to raised end diastolic pressure) but more often such disparities are due to other factors, such as the psychological state of the patient, their level of fitness or the demands which society makes on them. This is perhaps the strongest argument for an approach that, while recognising the importance of pathology and impairment, is targeted more directly at disability and handicap. A holistic approach to the patient requires consideration of all four elements – the integration of rehabilitation with medical and surgical management as described in the definition earlier.

Ask yourself whether your patient would be symptomatically better if he were fitter, whether he would be less distressed if he had a clearer understanding of his condition, whether managing his anxiety would improve his quality of life, or whether changing his behaviour might alter the natural history of his disease. If the answer to any of these is 'yes' then rehabilitation in some form should play a part in the management of his condition.

10.36 Who benefits most from cardiac rehabilitation?

Patients with new onset or resistant angina, recent myocardial infarction or recent coronary revascularisation benefit most from cardiac rehabilitation programmes.

In comparison to a sedentary lifestyle, regular physical activity is associated with approximately half the risk of future cardiac events. The benefits of regular exercise appear to relate, in part, to the associated

---

BOX 10.3 Rehabilitation

- *Pathology*: the disease process affecting the organ, such as coronary artery atheroma or valvular stenosis
- *Impairment*: the negative effect of the pathological process on the function of the organ, such as ischaemia, poor left ventricular function or low cardiac output
- *Disability*: the functional consequences of that impairment for the individual, such as loss of exercise tolerance or chest pain with emotion
- *Handicap*: the effects of that disability on the individual's role in society, such as unemployment, loss of status or having to give up golf

improvements in blood pressure and lipid profile. Most exercise programmes recommend at least 30 minutes of aerobic exercise three times a week.

The majority of randomised controlled trials of exercise programmes and cardiac rehabilitation have been conducted in patients who have sustained a recent myocardial infarction and indicate that significant morbidity and mortality benefits can be achieved. While the benefits appear to be most prominent in the first 2 years, the secondary preventative effects appear to be sustained over a 10-year period. However, these benefits were only seen when exercise is included as part of multiple lifestyle intervention programmes.

 PATIENT QUESTIONS

10.37 What is the best way of treating coronary heart disease?

There are many lifestyle changes that can treat coronary heart disease. The most important is stopping smoking. Continued smoking markedly increases the future risk of heart attacks and death. It is the single strongest 'risk factor' for future problems with coronary heart disease.

Regular exercise is good for the heart, especially when you have a heart condition. There may be some restrictions on activity but, in general, the more exercise you do, the better shape the heart will be in.

10.38 Is diet important?

Diet is extremely important. It is best to avoid dairy products including butter and cheese. These foods are high in animal fats and increase the risk of heart disease. A diet rich in fruit and vegetables and low in salt and saturated fats has been proven to reduce blood pressure and may well protect against heart disease. In addition, introducing oily fish into the diet and decreasing salt intake will also be of benefit in terms of blood pressure and reducing the risk of heart disease.

If you are overweight, it is sensible to lose weight as this decreases the strain on the heart as well as reducing blood pressure. It may also reduce the likelihood of developing 'sugar' diabetes, an important condition that increases the risk of coronary heart disease.

10.39 Is red wine good for the heart?

There is some evidence that drinking red wine in moderation (1–2 glasses per day) can reduce the risk of a heart attack. This could be due to an increase in the good (HDL) cholesterol. However, excessive alcohol intake, especially binge drinking, can increase blood pressure and increase the risk of coronary heart disease. The benefits of moderate alcohol intake are not restricted exclusively to red wine: other forms of alcohol, provided they are taken in moderation, may also be of benefit in protecting against coronary heart disease.

10.40 Is salt bad for the heart?

Increased salt (>7 g for men and >5 g for women) in the diet can cause an increase in blood pressure which is bad for the heart. For this reason doctors recommend moderate salt intake. In patients with increased blood pressure, it is especially important to keep salt intake low. Furthermore, it is important to recognise that there are 'hidden' levels of salt in many processed foods and ready-made meals and patients should read the labels on such products carefully to ascertain how much salt they contain.

APPENDIX
Useful addresses and websites

GP AND PATIENT INFORMATION

Blood Pressure Association
60 Cranmer Terrace
London SW17 0QS
Tel: 020 8772 4994
Fax: 020 8772 4999
www.bpassoc.org.uk

British Cardiac Patients Association
2 Station Road
Swavesey
Cambridge CB4 5QJ
Tel/fax: 01954 202022
Email:enquries@BCPA.co.uk
www.bcpa.co.uk

British Cardiac Society
9 Fitzroy Square
London W1T 5HW
Tel: 020 7383 3887
Fax: 020 7388 0903
www.bcs.com

British Heart Foundation
14 Fitzhardinge Street
London W1H 6DH
Tel: 020 7935 0185
Fax: 020 7486 5820
Email: internet@bhf.org.uk
www.bhf.org.uk

British Hypertension Society
Blood Pressure Unit, Department of Physiological Medicine
St George's Hospital Medical School
Cranmer Terrace
London SW17 0RE
Tel: 020 8725 3412
Fax: 020 8725 2959
Email: bhsis@sghms.ac.uk
www.hyp.ac.uk/bhs/

Coronary Prevention Group
2 Taviton Street
London WC1H 0BT
Tel: 020 7927 2125
Fax: 020 7927 2127
Email: cpg@lshtm.ac.uk
www.healthnet.org.uk

Family Heart Association
7 North Road
Maidenhead
Berkshire SL6 1PE
Tel: 01628 628638
Fax: 01628 628698
Email: md@familyheart.org
www.familyheart.org

National Heart Forum
Tavistock House South
Tavistock Square
London WC1H 9LG
Tel: 020 7383 7638
Fax: 020 7387 2779
Email: webenquiry@heartforum.org.uk
www.heartforum.org.uk/nationalheartforum.html

Primary Care Cardiovascular Society
36 Berrymede Road
London W4 5JD
Tel: 020 8994 8775
Fax: 020 8742 2130
Email: office@pccs.org.uk
www.pccs.org.uk

GOVERNMENT SITES AND GUIDELINES

- **CHMO site** (source of Chief Medical Officer's publications, including 'The Expert Patient') www.doh.gov.uk/cmo/publications.htm
- **Health Development Agency** (publications, including patient information sheets on heart disease, in Gujerati, Bengali, Hindi and Punjabi) www.hda-online.org.uk
- **National Heart, Lung & Blood Institute** (United States) (direct link to guide to lowering high blood pressure) www.nhlbi.nih.gov/hbp/index.html
- **NHS - Giving up smoking** www.givingupsmoking.co.uk
- **National Institute for Clinical Excellence** www.nice.org.uk
- **Scottish Intercollegiate Guidelines Network** (SIGN) www.sign.ac.uk
- **UK National Service Framework for Coronary Heart Disease (2000)** www.nelh.nhs.uk/nsf/chd/

RESEARCH

- **Canadian Cardiovascular Society** (journal-like website with information about cardiovascular research and resources in Canada) www.ccs.ca
- **CORDA** (The Coronary Artery Disease Research Association) www.corda.org.uk
- **Framingham Heart Study** (part of the National Heart, Lung & Blood Institute, USA, developed Framingham Heart Study Prediction Score Sheets) www.nhlbi.nih.gov/about/framingham/
- **Global Registry of Acute Coronary Events** (GRACE) www.umassmed.edu/outcomes/grace
- **National Heart Research Fund** www.heartresearch.org.uk
- **US National Institutes of Health** (biomedical research, free) www.health.nih.gov

INFORMATIVE WEBSITES FOR THE GP AND PATIENT

- **American College of Cardiology** www.acc.org
- **American Dietetic Association** www.eatright.org
- **American Heart Association** www.americanheart.org
- **BHF National Centre for Physical Activity and Health** www.bhfactive.org.uk
- **British Nutrition Foundation** www.nutrition.org.uk
- **European Society of Cardiology** www.escardio.org
- **Heart and Stroke Foundation of Canada** www.heartandstroke.ca
- **Heart Foundation** (Australia) www.heartfoundation.com.au
- **Heart Information Network** (US information website for patients) wwww.heartinfo.com
- **Irish Heart Foundation** www.irishheart.ie./happyheart

- **Lifeclinic** (patient website with links to blood pressure, diabetes, cholesterol and nutrition) www.lifeclinic.com
- **Medicine Net** (US website with patient information on common conditions, including high blood pressure) www.focusonhighbloodpressure.com
- **Mended Hearts, Inc** (US patient organisation) http://mendedhearts.org
- **Net Doctor** (UK patient information site) www.netdoctor.co.uk
- **QuitsmokingUK.com** (patient group) www.quitsmokinguk.com
- **US Food and Nutrition Information Center** www.nal.usda.gov/fnic/

JOURNALS

- Direct links are provided by www.cardiosource.com/library/journals to:
  American Heart Journal; American Journal of Cardiology; American Journal of Hypertension; Atherosclerosis; Evidence-Based Cardiovascular Medicine; International Journal of Cardiology; Journal of the American College of Cardiology; Lancet; Progess in Cardiovascular Diseases; Thrombosis Research; Trends in Cardiovascular Medicine
- *Blood Pressure Monitoring* www.bpmonitoring.com
- *British Medical Journal* http://bmj.bmjjournals.com
- *Cardiology in Review* www.cardiologyinreview.com
- *Circulation* http://circ.ahajournals.org
- *European Heart Journal* www.eurheartj.org
- *Heart* http://heart.bmjjournals.com
- *National Electronic Library for Health* (Specialist Library for Cardiovascular Diseases) http://rms.nelh.nhs.uk/cardiovascular
- *New England Journal of Medicine* www.nejm.org

REFERENCES

CHAPTER 1

1. Izzo J, Black HR (eds) Hypertension primer: the essentials of high blood pressure, 3rd edn. Philadelphia: Lippincott Williams & Wilkins, 2003.
2. Levi F, Lucchini F, Negri E, La Vecchia C. Trends in mortality from cardiovascular and cerebrovascular diseases in Europe and other areas of the world. *Heart* 2002;88:119–124.
3. Newby D, Grubb N. Cardiology – an illustrated colour text. Edinburgh: Churchill Livingstone, 2004.

CHAPTER 3

1. Luscher MS, Thygesen K, Ravkilde J, Heickendorff L. Applicability of cardiac troponin T and I for early risk stratification in unstable coronary artery disease. TRIM Study Group. Thrombin Inhibition in Myocardial ischemia. *Circulation* 1997;96(8):2578–2585.

CHAPTER 4

1. Haverkate F, Thompson SG, Pyke SD, Gallimore JR, Pepys MB. Production of C-reactive protein and risk of coronary events in stable and unstable angina. European Concerted Action on Thrombosis and Disabilities Angina Pectoris Study Group. *Lancet* 1997;349(9050):462–466.
2. Ridker PM, Rifai N, Rose L, Buring JE, Cook NR. Comparison of C-reactive protein and low-density lipoprotein cholesterol levels in the prediction of first cardiovascular events. *N Engl J Med* 2002;347:1557–1565.
3. Hackam DG, Anand SS. Emerging risk factors for atherosclerotic vascular disease: a critical review of the evidence. *JAMA* 2003;290(7):932–940.

CHAPTER 5

1. Ezzati M, Lopez AD, Rodgers A, Vander HS, Murray CJ. Selected major risk factors and global and regional burden of disease. *Lancet* 2002;360:1347–1360.
2. Murray CJ, Lauer JA, Hutubessy RC et al. Effectiveness and costs of interventions to lower systolic blood pressure and cholesterol: a global and regional analysis on reduction of cardiovascular-disease risk. *Lancet* 2003;361:717–725.
3. Heart Protection Study Collaborative Group. MRC/BHF Heart Protection Study of cholesterol lowering with simvastatin in 20,536 high-risk individuals: a randomised placebo-controlled trial. *Lancet* 2002;360:7–22.
4. Law MR, Wald NJ. Risk factor thresholds: their existence under scrutiny. *BMJ* 2002;324:1570–1576.
5. Izzo J, Black HR (eds) Hypertension primer: the essentials of high blood pressure, 3rd edn. Philadelphia: Lippincott Williams & Wilkins, 2003.
6. Vasan RS, Larson MG, Leip EP et al. Impact of high-normal blood pressure on the risk of cardiovascular disease. *N Engl J Med* 2001;345:1291–1297.
7. Franklin SS, Larson MG, Khan SA, Wong ND, Leip EP, Levy D. Does the relation of blood pressure to coronary heart disease risk change with aging? The Framingham Heart Study. *Circulation* 2001;103:1245–1249.
8. Sever P. Abandoning diastole: a personal view. *BMJ* 1999;318:1773.

9. O'Rourke MF, Gallagher DE. Pulse wave analysis. *J Hypertens* 1996;14:147–157.

10. Williams B, Poulter NR, Brown MJ et al and the BHS guidelines working party, for the British Hypertension Society. British Hypertension Society guidelines for hypertension management 2004 (BHS-IV): summary. *BMJ* 2004;328:634–640.

11. National Heart, Lung, and Blood Institute. Seventh Report of the Joint National Committee on prevention, detection, evaluation, and treatment of high blood pressure (JNC 7). Bethesda: NHLBI, 2003.

12. Haffner SM, Lehto S, Ronnemaa T, Pyorala K, Laakso M. Mortality from coronary heart disease in subjects with type 2 diabetes and in nondiabetic subjects with and without prior myocardial infarction. *N Engl J Med* 1998;339:229–234.

13. Collins R, Armitage J, Parish S, Sleigh P, Peto R. MRC/BHF Heart Protection Study of cholesterol-lowering with simvastatin in 5963 people with diabetes: a randomised placebo-controlled trial. *Lancet* 2003;361:2005–2016.

14. Gaede P, Vedel P, Larsen N, Jensen GV, Parving HH, Pedersen O. Multifactorial intervention and cardiovascular disease in patients with type 2 diabetes. *N Engl J Med* 2003;348:383–393.

15. Ornish D, Brown SE, Scherwitz LW et al. Can lifestyle changes reverse coronary heart disease? The Lifestyle Heart Trial. *Lancet* 1990;336:129–133.

16. Manson JE, Willett WC, Stampfer MJ et al. Body weight and mortality among women. *N Engl J Med* 1995;333:677–685.

17. Willett WC, Dietz WH, Colditz GA. Guidelines for healthy weight. *N Engl J Med* 1999;341:427–434.

18. Gronbaek M, Deis A, Sorensen TI, Becker U, Schnohr P, Jensen G. Mortality associated with moderate intakes of wine, beer, or spirits. *BMJ* 1995;310:1165–1169.

19. Sesso HD, Paffenbarger RS, Ha T, Lee IM. Physical activity and cardiovascular disease risk in middle-aged and older women. *Am J Epidemiol* 1999;150:408–416.

20. Wannamethee SG, Shaper AG, Walker M. Changes in physical activity, mortality, and incidence of coronary heart disease in older men. *Lancet* 1998;351:1603–1608.

21. Yu S, Yarnell JW, Sweetnam PM, Murray L. What level of physical activity protects against premature cardiovascular death? The Caerphilly study. *Heart* 2003;89:502–506.

22. Sesso HD, Paffenbarger RS Jr, Lee IM. Physical activity and coronary heart disease in men: The Harvard Alumni Health Study. *Circulation* 2000;102:975–980.

23. Oldridge NB, Guyatt GH, Fischer ME, Rimm AA. Cardiac rehabilitation after myocardial infarction. Combined experience of randomized clinical trials. *JAMA* 1988;260:945–950.

24. He J, Vupputuri S, Allen K, Prerost MR, Hughes J, Whelton PK. Passive smoking and the risk of coronary heart disease – a meta-analysis of epidemiologic studies. *N Engl J Med* 1999;340:920–926.

25. Blacher J, Guerin AP, Pannier B et al. Impact of aortic stiffness on survival in end-stage renal disease. *Circulation* 1999;99:2434–2439.

26. Blacher J, Safar ME, Guerin AP, Pannier B, Marchais SJ, London GM. Aortic pulse wave velocity index and mortality in end-stage renal disease. *Kidney Int* 2003;63:1852–1860.

27. Guerin AP, Blacher J, Pannier B, Marchais SJ, Safar ME, London GM.

Impact of aortic stiffness attenuation on survival of patients in end-stage renal failure. *Circulation* 2001;103:987–992.

CHAPTER 6

1. Juul-Moller S, Edvardsson N, Jahnmatz B, Rosen A, Sorensen S, Omblus R. Double-blind trial of aspirin in primary prevention of myocardial infarction in patients with stable chronic angina pectoris. The Swedish Angina Pectoris Aspirin Trial (SAPAT) Group. *Lancet* 1992;340:1421–1425.

2. Collaborative overview of randomised trials of antiplatelet therapy – I: Prevention of death, myocardial infarction, and stroke by prolonged antiplatelet therapy in various categories of patients. Antiplatelet Trialists' Collaboration. *BMJ* 1994;308:81–106.

3. Yusuf S, Sleight P, Pogue J, Bosch J, Davies R, Dagenais G. Effects of an angiotensin-converting-enzyme inhibitor, ramipril, on cardiovascular events in high-risk patients. The Heart Outcomes Prevention Evaluation Study Investigators. *N Engl J Med* 2000;342:145–153.

4. Fox KM. Efficacy of perindopril in reduction of cardiovascular events among patients with stable coronary artery disease: randomised, double-blind, placebo-controlled, multicentre trial (the EUROPA study). *Lancet* 2003;362:782–788.

5. Held P, Yusuf S. Early intravenous beta-blockade in acute myocardial infarction. *Cardiology* 1989;76:132–143.

6. Savonitto S, Ardissiono D, Egstrup K et al. Combination therapy with metoprolol and nifedipine versus monotherapy in patients with stable angina pectoris. Results of the International Multicenter Angina Exercise (IMAGE) Study. *J Am Coll Cardiol* 1996;27:311–316.

7. Heidenreich PA, McDonald KM, Hastie T, Fadel B, Hagan V, Lee BK, Hlatky MA. Meta-analysis of trials comparing beta-blockers, calcium antagonists, and nitrates for stable angina. *JAMA* 1999;281:1927–1936.

8. Psaty BM, Heckbert SR, Koepsell TD et al. The risk of myocardial infarction associated with antihypertensive drug therapies. *JAMA* 1995;274:620–625.

9. Furberg CD, Psaty BM, Meyer JV. Nifedipine. Dose-related increase in mortality in patients with coronary heart disease. *Circulation* 1995;92:1326–1331.

10. Effect of nicorandil on coronary events in patients with stable angina: the impact of nicorandil in angina (IONA) randomised trial. *Lancet* 2002;359:1269–1275.

11. The European Stroke Prevention Study (ESPS). Principal end-points. The ESPS Group. *Lancet* 1987;2:1351–1354.

12. A randomised, blinded, trial of clopidogrel versus aspirin in patients at risk of ischaemic events (CAPRIE). CAPRIE Steering Committee. *Lancet* 1996;348:1329–1339.

13. Peters RJ, Mehta SR, Fox KA et al. Effects of aspirin dose when used alone or in combination with clopidogrel in patients with acute coronary syndromes: observations from the clopidogrel in unstable angina to prevent recurrent events (CURE) study. *Circulation* 2003;108:1682–1687.

14. Kugiyama K, Motoyama T, Hirashima O et al. Vitamin C attenuates abnormal vasomotor reactivity in spasm coronary arteries in patients with coronary spastic angina. *J Am Coll Cardiol* 1998;32:103–109.

15. Stephens NG, Parsons A, Schofield PM, Kelly F, Cheeseman K,

Mitchinson MJ. Randomised controlled trial of vitamin E in patients with coronary disease: Cambridge Heart Antioxidant Study (CHAOS). *Lancet* 1996;347:781–786.

16. Kamikawa T, Kobayashi A, Yamashita T, Hayashi H, Yamazaki N. Effects of coenzyme Q10 on exercise tolerance in chronic stable angina pectoris. *Am J Cardiol* 1985;56:247–251.

17. Yusuf S, Dagenais G, Pogue J, Bosch J, Sleight P. Vitamin E supplementation and cardiovascular events in high-risk patients. The Heart Outcomes Prevention Evaluation Study Investigators. *N Engl J Med* 2000;342:154–160.

18. Maxwell AJ, Zapien MP, Pearce GL, MacCallum G, Stone PH. Randomized trial of a medical food for the dietary management of chronic, stable angina. *J Am Coll Cardiol* 2002;39:37–45.

19. Wright RS, Murphy JG, Bybee KA, Kopecky SL, LaBlanche JM. Statin lipid-lowering therapy for acute myocardial infarction and unstable angina: efficacy and mechanism of benefit. *Mayo Clin Proc* 2002;77:1085–1092.

20. Fathi R, Haluska B, Short L, Marwick TH. A randomized trial of aggressive lipid reduction for improvement of myocardial ischemia, symptom status, and vascular function in patients with coronary artery disease not amenable to intervention. *Am J Med* 2003;114:445–453.

21. Burr ML, Fehily AM, Gilbert JF et al. Effects of changes in fat, fish, and fibre intakes on death and myocardial reinfarction: diet and reinfarction trial (DART). *Lancet* 1989;2:757–761.

22. Dietary supplementation with n-3 polyunsaturated fatty acids and vitamin E after myocardial infarction: results of the GISSI-Prevenzione trial. Gruppo Italiano per lo Studio della Sopravvivenza nell'Infarto miocardico. *Lancet* 1999;354:447–455.

23. Burr ML, Ashfield-Watt PA, Dunstan FD et al. Lack of benefit of dietary advice to men with angina: results of a controlled trial. *Eur J Clin Nutr* 2003;57:193–200.

24. Dwyer JH, Allayee H, Dwyer KM et al. Arachidonate 5-lipoxygenase promoter genotype, dietary arachidonic acid, and atherosclerosis. *N Engl J Med* 2004;350:29–37.

25. Kris-Etherton PM, Harris WS, Appel LJ. Fish consumption, fish oil, omega-3 fatty acids, and cardiovascular disease. *Circulation* 2002;106:2747–2757.

CHAPTER 7

1. Keeley EC, Boura JA, Grines CL. Primary angioplasty versus intravenous thrombolytic therapy for acute myocardial infarction: a quantitative review of 23 randomised trials. *Lancet* 2003;361:13–20.

2. Moses JW, Leon MB, Popma JJ et al. Sirolimus-eluting stents versus standard stents in patients with stenosis in a native coronary artery. *N Engl J Med* 2003;349:1315–1323.

3. Coronary angioplasty versus medical therapy for angina: the second Randomised Intervention Treatment of Angina (RITA-2) trial. RITA-2 trial participants. *Lancet* 1997;350:461–468.

4. Parisi AF, Folland ED, Hartigan P. A comparison of angioplasty with medical therapy in the treatment of single-vessel coronary artery disease. Veterans Affairs ACME Investigators. *N Engl J Med* 1992;326:10–16.

5. de Bono D. Complications of diagnostic cardiac catheterisation: results from 34,041 patients in the United Kingdom confidential enquiry

into cardiac catheter complications. The Joint Audit Committee of the British Cardiac Society and Royal College of Physicians of London. *Br Heart J* 1993;70:297–300.

6. Smith SC, Jr, Dove JT, Jacobs AK et al. ACC/AHA guidelines of percutaneous coronary interventions (revision of the 1993 PTCA guidelines) – executive summary. A report of the American College of Cardiology/American Heart Association Task Force on Practice Guidelines (committee to revise the 1993 guidelines for percutaneous transluminal coronary angioplasty). *J Am Coll Cardiol* 2001;37:2215–2239.

7. Steinhubl SR, Berger PB, Mann JT et al. Early and sustained dual oral antiplatelet therapy following percutaneous coronary intervention: a randomized controlled trial. *JAMA* 2002;288:2411–2420.

8. Coronary artery bypass surgery versus percutaneous coronary intervention with stent implantation in patients with multivessel coronary artery disease (the Stent or Surgery trial): a randomised controlled trial. *Lancet* 2002;360:965–970.

9. Pocock SJ, Henderson RA, Rickards AF et al. Meta-analysis of randomised trials comparing coronary angioplasty with bypass surgery. *Lancet* 1995;346:1184–1189.

10. Comparison of coronary bypass surgery with angioplasty in patients with multivessel disease. The Bypass Angioplasty Revascularization Investigation (BARI) Investigators. *N Engl J Med* 1996;335:217–225.

CHAPTER 8

1. Peters RJ, Mehta SR, Fox KA et al. Effects of aspirin dose when used alone or in combination with clopidogrel in patients with acute coronary syndromes: observations from the Clopidogrel in Unstable angina to prevent Recurrent Events (CURE) study. *Circulation* 2003;108:1682–1687.

2. Braunwald E, Antman EM, Beasley JW et al. ACC/AHA guideline update for the management of patients with unstable angina and non-ST-segment elevation myocardial infarction – 2002. Summary article: a report of the American College of Cardiology/American Heart Association Task Force on Practice Guidelines (Committee on the Management of Patients With Unstable Angina). *Circulation* 2002;106:1893–1900.

3. Collaborative overview of randomised trials of antiplatelet therapy – I: Prevention of death, myocardial infarction, and stroke by prolonged antiplatelet therapy in various categories of patients. Antiplatelet Trialists' Collaboration. *BMJ* 1994;308:81–106.

4. Boersma E, Harrington RA, Moliterno DJ et al. Platelet glycoprotein IIb/IIIa inhibitors in acute coronary syndromes: a meta-analysis of all major randomised clinical trials. *Lancet* 2002;359:189–198.

5. Fox KA, Antman EM, Cohen M, Bigonzi F. Comparison of enoxaparin versus unfractionated heparin in patients with unstable angina pectoris/non-ST-segment elevation acute myocardial infarction having subsequent percutaneous coronary intervention. *Am J Cardiol* 2002;90:477–482.

6. Metz BK, White HD, Granger CB et al. Randomized comparison of direct thrombin inhibition versus heparin in conjunction with fibrinolytic therapy for acute myocardial infarction: results from the GUSTO-IIb Trial. Global Use

of Strategies to Open Occluded Coronary Arteries in Acute Coronary Syndromes (GUSTO-IIb) Investigators. *J Am Coll Cardiol* 1998;31:1493–1498.

7. Indications for fibrinolytic therapy in suspected acute myocardial infarction: collaborative overview of early mortality and major morbidity results from all randomised trials of more than 1000 patients. Fibrinolytic Therapy Trialists' (FTT) Collaborative Group. *Lancet* 1994;343:311–322.

8. Opie LH, Yusuf S, Kubler W. Current status of safety and efficacy of calcium channel blockers in cardiovascular diseases: a critical analysis based on 100 studies. *Prog Cardiovasc Dis* 2000;43:171–196.

9. Granger CB, Goldberg RJ, Dabbous O et al. Global Registry of Acute Coronary Events Investigators. Predictors of hospital mortality in the global registry of acute coronary events. *Arch Intern Med* 2003;163(19):2345–2353.

10. Boden WE, O'Rourke RA, Crawford MH et al. Outcomes in patients with acute non-Q-wave myocardial infarction randomly assigned to an invasive as compared with a conservative management strategy. Veterans Affairs Non-Q-Wave Infarction Strategies in Hospital (VANQWISH) Trial Investigators. *N Engl J Med* 1998;338:1785–1792.

11. Invasive compared with non-invasive treatment in unstable coronary-artery disease: FRISC II prospective randomised multicentre study. FRagmin and Fast Revascularisation during InStability in Coronary artery disease Investigators. *Lancet* 1999;354:708–715.

12. Cannon CP, Weintraub WS, Demopoulos LA et al. Comparison of early invasive and conservative strategies in patients with unstable coronary syndromes treated with the glycoprotein IIb/IIIa inhibitor tirofiban. *N Engl J Med* 2001;344:1879–1887.

13. Fox KA, Poole-Wilson PA, Henderson RA et al. Interventional versus conservative treatment for patients with unstable angina or non-ST-elevation myocardial infarction: the British Heart Foundation RITA-3 randomised trial. Randomized Intervention Trial of unstable Angina. *Lancet* 2002;360:743–751.

CHAPTER 9

1. Randomised trial of intravenous streptokinase, oral aspirin, both, or neither among 17,187 cases of suspected acute myocardial infarction: ISIS-2. ISIS-2 (Second International Study of Infarct Survival) Collaborative Group. *Lancet* 1988;2:349–360.

2. Topol EJ. Reperfusion therapy for acute myocardial infarction with fibrinolytic therapy or combination reduced fibrinolytic therapy and platelet glycoprotein IIb/IIIa inhibition: the GUSTO V randomised trial. *Lancet* 2001;357:1905–1914.

3. Indications for fibrinolytic therapy in suspected acute myocardial infarction: collaborative overview of early mortality and major morbidity results from all randomised trials of more than 1000 patients. Fibrinolytic Therapy Trialists' (FTT) Collaborative Group. *Lancet* 1994;343:311–322.

4. ISIS-3: a randomised comparison of streptokinase vs tissue plasminogen activator vs anistreplase and of aspirin plus heparin vs aspirin alone among 41,299 cases of suspected acute myocardial infarction. ISIS-3 (Third

International Study of Infarct Survival) Collaborative Group. *Lancet* 1992;339:753–770.

5. An international randomized trial comparing four thrombolytic strategies for acute myocardial infarction. The GUSTO investigators. *N Engl J Med* 1993;329:673–682.

6. Feasibility, safety, and efficacy of domiciliary thrombolysis by general practitioners: Grampian region early anistreplase trial. GREAT Group. *BMJ* 1992;305:548–553.

7. Keeley EC, Boura JA, Grines CL. Primary angioplasty versus intravenous thrombolytic therapy for acute myocardial infarction: a quantitative review of 23 randomised trials. *Lancet* 2003;361:13–20.

8. Randomised trial of intravenous atenolol among 16 027 cases of suspected acute myocardial infarction: ISIS-1. First International Study of Infarct Survival Collaborative Group. *Lancet* 1986;2:57–66.

9. Comparison of invasive and conservative strategies after treatment with intravenous tissue plasminogen activator in acute myocardial infarction. Results of the thrombolysis in myocardial infarction (TIMI) phase II trial. The TIMI Study Group. *N Engl J Med* 1989;320:618–627.

10. Indications for ACE inhibitors in the early treatment of acute myocardial infarction: systematic overview of individual data from 100,000 patients in randomized trials. ACE Inhibitor Myocardial Infarction Collaborative Group. *Circulation* 1998;97:2202–2212.

CHAPTER 10

1. Collaborative overview of randomised trials of antiplatelet therapy – I: Prevention of death, myocardial infarction, and stroke by prolonged antiplatelet therapy in various categories of patients. Antiplatelet Trialists' Collaboration. *BMJ* 1994;308:81–106.

2. Rang HP, Dale MM, Ritter JM, Moore P (eds) Pharmacology, 5th edn. Edinburgh: Churchill Livingstone, 2003.

3. Comparison of sibrafiban with aspirin for prevention of cardiovascular events after acute coronary syndromes: a randomised trial. The SYMPHONY Investigators. Sibrafiban versus Aspirin to Yield Maximum Protection from Ischemic Heart Events Post-acute Coronary Syndromes. *Lancet* 2000;355:337–345.

4. Randomized trial of aspirin, sibrafiban, or both for secondary prevention after acute coronary syndromes. *Circulation* 2001;103:1727–1733.

5. Anand SA, Yusuf S. Oral anticoagulants in patients with coronary artery disease. *J Am Coll Cardiol* 2003;41:62S–69S.

6. Scandinavian Simvastatin Survival Study Group. Randomized trial of cholesterol lowering in 4444 patients with coronary heart disease: the Scandinavian Simvastatin Survival Study (4S). *Lancet* 1995;344:1383–1389.

7. MRC/BHF Heart Protection Study of cholesterol lowering with simvastatin in 20,536 high-risk individuals: a randomised placebo-controlled trial. *Lancet* 2002;360:7–22.

8. Schwartz GG, Olsson AG, Ezekowitz MD. Effects of atorvastatin on early recurrent ischemic events in acute coronary syndromes: the MIRACL study: a randomized controlled trial. *JAMA* 2001;285:1711–1718.

9. Rubins HB, Robins SJ, Collins D et al. Gemfibrozil for the secondary prevention of coronary heart disease in men with low levels of high-density

lipoprotein cholesterol. Veterans Affairs High-Density Lipoprotein Cholesterol Intervention Trial Study Group. *N Engl J Med* 1999;341:410–418.

10. Freemantle N, Cleland J, Young P, Mason J, Harrison J. Beta blockade after myocardial infarction: systematic review and meta regression analysis. *BMJ* 1999;318:1730–1737.

11. Poole-Wilson PA, Swedberg K, Cleland JG et al. Comparison of carvedilol and metoprolol on clinical outcomes in patients with chronic heart failure in the Carvedilol Or Metoprolol European Trial (COMET): randomised controlled trial. *Lancet* 2003;362:7–13.

12. Yusuf S, Sleight P, Pogue J, Bosch J, Davies R, Dagenais G. Effects of an angiotensin-converting-enzyme inhibitor, ramipril, on cardiovascular events in high-risk patients. The Heart Outcomes Prevention Evaluation Study Investigators. *N Engl J Med* 2000;342:145–153.

13. Fox KM. Efficacy of perindopril in reduction of cardiovascular events among patients with stable coronary artery disease: randomised, double-blind, placebo-controlled, multicentre trial (the EUROPA study). *Lancet* 2003;362:782–788.

14. Flather MD, Yusuf S, Kober L et al. Long-term ACE-inhibitor therapy in patients with heart failure or left-ventricular dysfunction: a systematic overview of data from individual patients. ACE-Inhibitor Myocardial Infarction Collaborative Group. *Lancet* 2000;355:1575–1581.

15. Pitt B, Segal R, Martinez FA et al. Randomised trial of losartan versus captopril in patients over 65 with heart failure (Evaluation of Losartan in the Elderly Study, ELITE). *Lancet* 1997;349:747–752.

16. Pitt B, Poole-Wilson PA, Segal R et al. Effect of losartan compared with captopril on mortality in patients with symptomatic heart failure: randomised trial – the Losartan Heart Failure Survival Study ELITE II. *Lancet* 2000;355:1582–1587.

17. Dickstein K, Kjekshus J. Comparison of baseline data, initial course, and management: losartan versus captopril following acute myocardial infarction (The OPTIMAAL Trial). OPTIMAAL Trial Steering Committee and Investigators. Optimal Trial in Myocardial Infarction with the Angiotensin II Antagonist Losartan. *Am J Cardiol* 2001;87:766–771, A7.

18. Yusuf S, Pfeffer MA, Swedberg K et al. Effects of candesartan in patients with chronic heart failure and preserved left-ventricular ejection fraction: the CHARM-Preserved Trial. *Lancet* 2003;362:777–781.

19. Hulley S, Grady D, Bush T et al. Randomized trial of estrogen plus progestin for secondary prevention of coronary heart disease in postmenopausal women. Heart and Estrogen/progestin Replacement Study (HERS) Research Group. *JAMA* 1998;280:605–613.

20. Hodis HN, Mack WJ, Azen SP et al. Hormone therapy and the progression of coronary-artery atherosclerosis in postmenopausal women. *N Engl J Med* 2003;349:535–545.

21. Rossouw JE, Anderson GL, Prentice RL et al. Risks and benefits of estrogen plus progestin in healthy postmenopausal women: principal results from the Women's Health Initiative randomized controlled trial. *JAMA* 2002;288:321–333.

22. Stephens NG, Parsons A, Schofield PM et al. Randomised controlled trial of vitamin E in patients with coronary disease: Cambridge Heart Antioxidant

Study (CHAOS). *Lancet* 1996;347:781–786.

23. Vivekananthan DP, Penn MS, Sapp SK, Hsu A, Topol EJ. Use of antioxidant vitamins for the prevention of cardiovascular disease: meta-analysis of randomised trials. *Lancet* 2003;361:2017–2023.

24. Burr ML, Fehily AM, Gilbert JF et al. Effects of changes in fat, fish, and fibre intakes on death and myocardial reinfarction: diet and reinfarction trial (DART). *Lancet* 1989;2:757–761.

25. Dietary supplementation with n-3 polyunsaturated fatty acids and vitamin E after myocardial infarction: results of the GISSI-Prevenzione trial. Gruppo Italiano per lo Studio della Sopravvivenza nell'Infarto miocardico. *Lancet* 1999;354:447–455.

LIST OF PATIENT QUESTIONS

INDEX

Note: Abbreviations: CHD, Coronary heart disease; MI, Myocardial infarction
As coronary heart disease is the subject of this book, all index entries refer to coronary heart disease unless otherwise indicated.
Page numbers in **bold** refer to figures/tables/boxes.

D

E

S

U

V

W

X

Z